Become Extraordinary

Janelle Ryan

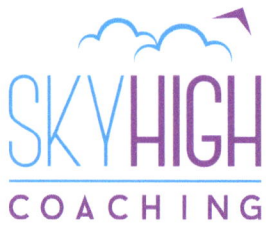

First published by Busybird Publishing 2020

Copyright © 2020 Janelle Ryan

Print: 978-1-922465-33-7
Ebook: 978-1-922465-34-4

This work is copyright. Apart from any use permitted under the *Copyright Act 1968*, no part of this publication may be reproduced, stored in a retrieval system or transmitted in any form or by any means, electronic, mechanical, photocopying, recording or otherwise, without the prior written permission of Janelle Ryan.

Cover Image: Natalie Rowe
Cover design: Busybird Publishing
Layout and typesetting: Busybird Publishing
Illustrations: Kev Howlett

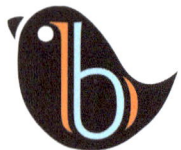

Busybird Publishing
2/118 Para Road
Montmorency, Victoria
Australia 3094

*This book is dedicated to four extraordinary women:
Glenys Farley, Jean Farley, Mavis Wake
and Marjorie Molloy.*

Praise for
BECOME EXTRAORDINARY

'A powerful book that gives you practical steps towards achieving what seems to be impossible. Your life begins at the end of these chapters.'
Lisa Cavill
Company Director

'If you are ready to 'get unstuck' and smash through some 'stuff' that is holding you back in any area of your life then I highly recommend this book.'
Wendy Barron
Personal Trainer & Lifestyle Coach

'Janelle Ryan has had such a deep impact on my life. Without her coaching approach I wouldn't be where I am today. If you are looking for practical tips that will support your growth and learning, Janelle Ryan's got them!'
Stephanie Abouatallah
Founder of BlueHiveHealth.com and Senior Account Executive

'Janelle brings a practical down-to-earth approach to some of the deepest and most existential issues we face; least of which, 'what is my purpose?"
Giovanna Capozza
Relationship Coach, Spiritual Teacher, Speaker and International Retreat Leader

'Since working with Janelle I have become calmer, stronger and more resilient. My emotional intelligence has grown in a way I hadn't anticipated and external situations and people no longer have the ability to raise unwanted emotions in me. Every chapter in this book gives you powerful tools and activities. Work through them and your life will transform.'
Sidonie Berke
Lawyer

'Consciously creating the life of your dreams starts right here, with empowering and practical strategies that actually work! Janelle's passion and authenticity jump out of every page and pull you in (with both hands) equipping you with the confidence to know that if you do the work, you *will* get results. Prepare to be inspired.'
Nikki Karpeles
Public Relations and Communications Professional

Contents

Foreword	i
Introduction	iii
Clarify Your Vision	1
Bring Your Vision to Life	15
Unwrap Your Gifts	25
Smash Through Self-Doubt	35
Create More Confidence	49
Raise Your Resilience	65
Tame The Treadmill	77
Make Friends With Fear	89
Take A Quantum Leap	103
Acknowledgements	129
About The Author	133

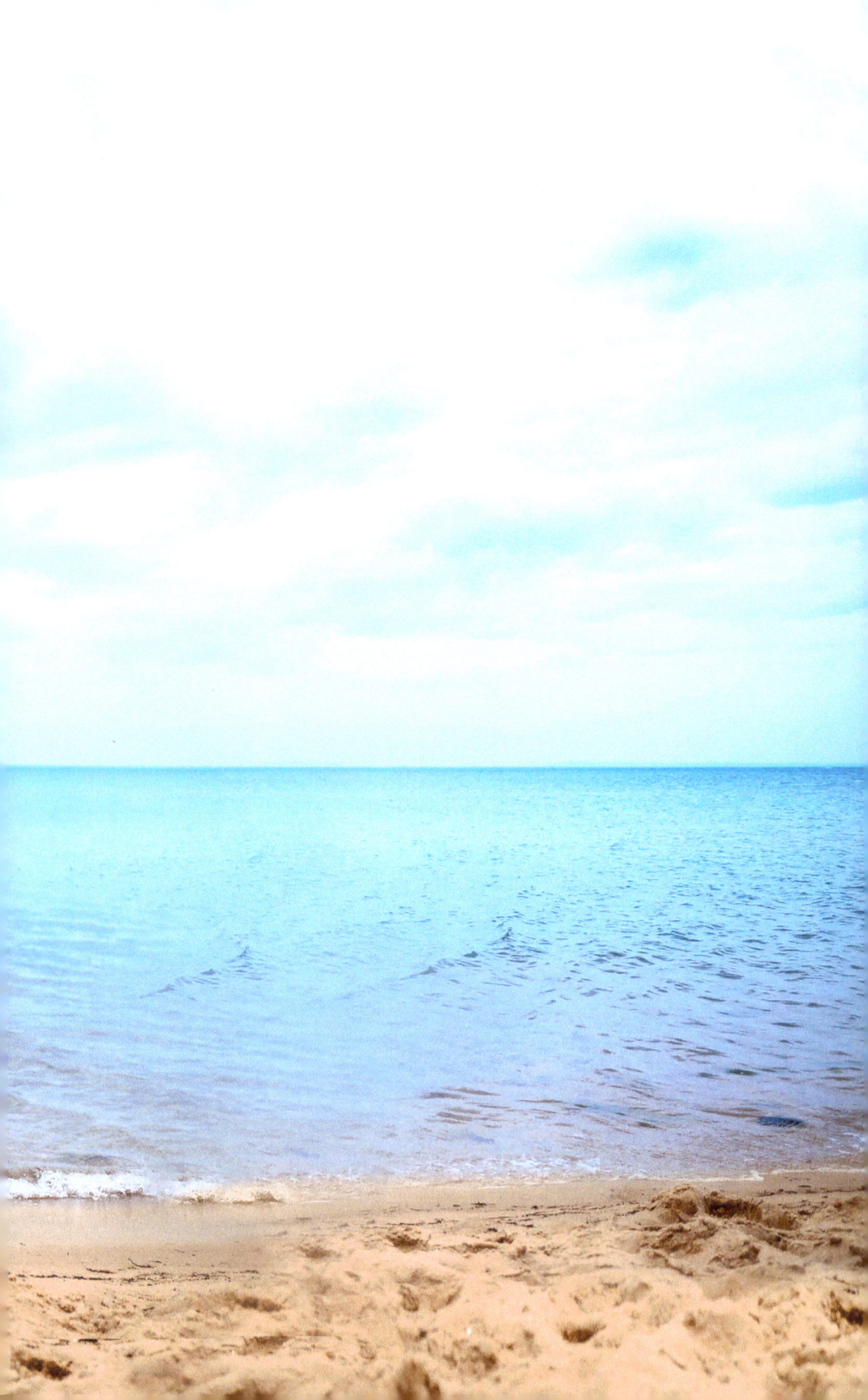

Foreword

by Kate James

Coach, meditation teacher, speaker and writer

Janelle's main purpose and passion is to make a difference – to help others see how extraordinary and limitless they are, and to show them how to create a life that is the most fulfilling one it can be.

She is a shining example of someone who has done this herself. Through seeking help, challenging her mindset and changing her behaviour, she overcame her fears and discovered her own version of a meaningful life. Janelle has been *you*.

I first met Janelle in the early 2000s when she approached me for coaching. She had recently returned to Australia after residing in Europe for many years, and was unsure how to create a new life for herself in Melbourne. We spent six months together and during that time I watched as Janelle embraced coaching principles and tools, and used them to lay a foundation for her future. Before long she had designed a vision for her life that aligned with her values. Janelle took responsibility for her own transformation by turning inwards and examining her own beliefs, attitudes and behaviours, even when she was afraid to. A few years after our coaching program, Janelle had completed a university degree, stepped into a dream job and saved a deposit to buy her first home.

A true advocate of the coaching process, Janelle returned to me a few years later when she was ready for a leadership role, which she achieved within months. She returned again eight years after that, when she had become disillusioned with corporate life and was ready to make change. She wanted to build something of her own; she just wasn't sure what that was.

It became apparent very quickly, via values, skills, strengths and personality testing, that coaching was Janelle's most aligned vocation. Within eighteen months she received formal qualifications and launched Sky High Coaching. Within six months of the launch she left her full-time corporate role to devote her time to her clients and her business.

If you are looking for a book that is simple in its delivery; contains personal stories from the author who has lived through her own transformation (which wasn't always easy) and has a life-long passion for learning; outlines the theory behind the concepts in a way that's easy to understand; provides effective activities and exercises to work through and implement to create immediate change; is supported by real-life client case studies; and shows how you, and your life, can become truly extraordinary, then this is the book for you.

I hope you enjoy it.

Introduction

extraordinary:

1. unusual or remarkable

2. usually great

Anaïs Nin once wrote, 'We do not see things as they are, we see things as we are.' Do you see yourself as the extraordinary person you are, understand the power and energy at your disposal every moment of every day? Do you know the magnitude of what had to take place on a physical, mystical and spiritual level for you to be here on Earth? Do you know, at a deeply fundamental level, that you have the capability, skills and talent to create anything you wish?

Perpetually curious and a passionate pupil, I have spent decades diving into why I think, feel and behave the way I do. I've wondered why I'm here, and what my place is within the Universal landscape. I've wondered how to tap into the unseen forces at work around me (upon discovering they existed), and how to use them to my advantage. Am I truly the powerful creator of my own world, or is my fate at the whim of other people and external circumstances and events?

This lifelong endeavour has taken me around the world, exposing me to cutting edge scientific and spiritual concepts, introduced and delivered by some of the most brilliant minds today. Veils have been lifted, onion layers peeled back and truths revealed. It's been a very long road, but not by any means complete.

When I reflect over my life I can now clearly see I spent not years, but decades creating my world when I had no idea *how* I was doing it. Actually, to be honest I had no idea I *was* doing it. Like most people, I moved through life assuming life would happen *to* me, and I'd navigate through it to the best of my ability. I thought my role, when it came to the creation of my life, was to have some goals and take the conventional step-by-step approach to reach them. If something tripped me up along the way I usually blamed life, others, or myself (*if only I'd been born richer or thinner or smarter or funnier, with longer legs, or in a different city or country … if only I'd made Choice X instead of Choice Y … you know the drill …*)

Like most people, I thought I'd be happy when I reached the next goal, then the next. My happiness was linked to external factors which, I'm sure you'll agree, is not soul-fulfilling or inner happiness.

But twenty years ago something happened. I stopped dabbling in this 'self-help area' that I'd always loved and started studying mind-mastery; mastery of the dynamic of our two levels of mind – the conscious and subconscious. I mixed in some study of natural laws, spiritual laws, physics and universal energy, and everything changed for me. I learned how to consciously create anything at any time, and I was recently deemed to be in the top 6% happiest people on the planet.

We live in one of the most exciting times in history, as science and spirituality is coming together like never before. It's particularly thrilling for me because, as a deeply spiritual person, I am incredibly open to laws and theories that exist on a metaphysical plane, but as a practical down-to-earth Capricorn, I love a bit of science! I want to know how it works.

So with me, you're getting both sides of the story.

In this book I've included my knowledge, experiences, failures and successes with you. I will introduce you to what may appear unconventional phenomena, then pivot into some scientific facts.

The experiences I speak of are my own and are very personal to me. I have included client case studies; their names are fictitious to protect their privacy. This does not mean they will be your experiences; they are merely some of our examples.

This book is not designed to be read once and popped back onto your bookshelf. It's a working template, a journal, a notebook to be written on, scribbled in and referred back to for many years to come. It contains coaching tools and techniques which I encourage you to use and reuse over time. If you'd like additional resources and worksheets they can be found at my website **www.skyhighcoaching.com.au** and are absolutely my gift to you.

As you expand your mind and up level your life, these tools continue to remain relevant. The case studies included in this book illustrate the long term success that can be achieved with a handful of coaching tools.

Long term transformational change is just as it's described: long term. Make a commitment to yourself, right here and now, that you will read every word and complete every activity until you see a tangible, positive change in your life – in other words, for as long as it takes.

Some of these activities will amuse you, some may seem irrelevant, and others will challenge you. Have a giggle (life is supposed to be fun), put aside what doesn't serve you, dive boldly into what does and stay the course. It will be worth it.

My commitment to you is that I will be here for your whole adventure. I will prove to you how extraordinary and powerful you are. I will show you how to remove voices of doubt, make friends with fear, ooze poise and confidence (even when you're not particularly feeling it), rebuild your resilience and harness your energy. I will teach you how to uncover the hidden skills, strengths and gifts you didn't know you had. I will introduce you to the unseen forces at work around you and show you how to use them to your advantage. By the end of these pages you will know how to create your world from the inside out and become the master of your mind and your life – with elegance, grace and ease.

I will show you how extraordinary your life can be.

Are you ready?

Clarify Your Vision

'Since I have become clear on what I need and want, all aspects of my life have benefited.'

– Madeline, Extraordinary Client

In the year 2000, after almost five years exploring a rather large patch of the globe, I returned to Australia from my overseas adventure. After disembarking from the very long flight, like many before me I sought refuge in my parents' home. For many weeks I enjoyed reconnecting with family, home-cooked meals, being pampered, being able to shower without wearing thongs (or flip flops, depending on where you're from), and having a washing machine *inside* the home – one that I could use whenever I liked!

Within six weeks of gracing them with my presence, my parents started dropping subtle hints towards my departure. Initial words and phrases – such as *'job'* and *'completing your university degree'* popped up, quickly followed by *'when are you going to leave?'* and *'we are enjoying being empty nesters, you know'* – reminded me that the next chapter of my life was tapping at the front door. Literally! These faint whisperings had extended to clandestine phone calls to my best friend, who appeared on my parents' doorstep one day, hurled my repacked backpack *(how did that happen?)* into her car and escorted me back to the big smoke of Melbourne.

So there I was, bunking in my friend's spare room (for which I am eternally grateful) without a job, money or qualifications of any kind. I was overweight, unfit, unhealthy and a little discombobulated in my new surroundings. I was also heartbroken after a particularly painful breakup. I had no idea who I was, what I wanted in my life (or career) or what to do next. Feelings of displacement rendered me unable to commit to a job, a rental lease on a home or a return to university. I started some temporary work assignments, paid my friend some board money and wondered what I would be when I grew up. There was no clarity around what I wanted to create in my life or my career.

I knew I needed help and sought assistance from the first life coach I'd ever met, who I refer to as Beautiful Kate. The work we did together felt like magic and within six months I was well on the way to consciously creating the life of my dreams.

Looking back over my life, I can now see how envious I was of the people I knew who had *aspirations!* You know those people – the ones who have always known what they wanted to do. The dedicated classmates with future university courses selected, intended to launch them into fulfilling careers. Sporting teammates dreaming of representing Australia. The teen actors starring in the school musical whilst auditioning for professional acting roles. The friends who looked forward to creating their own family and children. The adventurers I met on my travels who knew exactly when they were returning home and exactly what they were going to do when they arrived!

I never understood the importance of clarity. My life had been a series of events thrown together at whatever whim I entertained that week, month or year. Ideas were plenty, and some eventuated, but I considered that to be nothing but wonderful coincidence, good timing or a helping hand extended by someone else. My life was one of *unconscious creation*, or you may know it as 'flying by the seat of my pants' ... that is until the year 2000, when I met my first coach, Kate.

Your being here on Earth is no accident. A LOT had to happen for you to be born. Ask anyone who's struggled with conception (oh yes, that was me). Birth is such a miracle – so many stars have to align – that it is truly a wonder any of us are here at all! I had always believed, long before I was a coach, that we are all here for a reason. Are you a little fuzzy right now on what yours is? You are not alone.

Remember when you were a child and the possibilities were endless? We wanted to be astronauts, superheroes and sports stars ... we didn't give ourselves any limits. We knew instinctively we didn't have to. We understood, at a cellular level, that we were limitless.

But sometimes, during our adventure into adulthood, we forget we still have imagination. We still have dreams. We still have desires that burn inside us ... and those dreams are *still possible*. They may not come in their original packaging. They may not look exactly as you thought they would. They may be in a different format. But, if they are right for you, they will *feel* just as exhilarating. If you have an idea, dream, desire or vision that keeps coming up, I encourage you to *pay attention*. It's popping up for a reason, and is probably not going to leave anytime soon.

Maybe you feel as though you've never had clarity around a vision for your life – or you had a clear vision, achieved it, and feel a bit stuck on what you'd like to create next. Maybe you have a vision that feels uncomfortable; it almost feels like something you *should* do, rather than something you *want* to do. Maybe you have a vision that feels so unaligned, you've realised it's a vision someone else held for you and you've accepted it as your own. Or maybe you have *kind of an idea* of something you'd love to create, but you're just not sure it's for you.

To move from an *unconsciously created* life into a *consciously created* life, your vision must be crystal clear. It doesn't necessarily have to be something that will change the world, but feel free if that's what comes up – I won't stop you. The only person it has to mean something to, the only person who has to feel in alignment with it, is you!

You don't have to know how you are going to get there, but believe me, you have to know what *there* looks like. It has to have texture, soul, colour, sound and scent. It has to unleash your tears, keep you awake at night, light up your soul, fire up your spirit and cause your entire body to vibrate with energy! It's your fuel, your light, your calling. Even if you won the major lottery tomorrow, you would *still* be driven to do this.

How do you tap into your truest desires? The ones your soul is patiently waiting for you to discover? Let's dive in.

ACTIVITY

Step 1

Grab something to write with – coloured pens are great for this. Got kids? Feel free to raid their pencil cases.

Step 2

Find a quiet place you will not be disturbed for at least an hour.

Step 3

Write your overarching heading – VISION.

Underneath, create some columns that represent the major areas of your life. Some to choose from include romantic life/partner, career, education, friendships, family, health, fitness, emotional health, purpose, spirituality, finances. Or create your own.

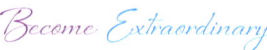

Clarify Your Vision

Step 4

If you are familiar and confident in slowing down and connecting to your intuition/ guides/ spirit/ soul/ God/ Universe (whatever the correct word is for you), please go ahead and do that now.

Alternatively, if this is a brand new experience for you, perfect! Let's play. Close your eyes and allow your breath to become slower and deeper. Relax your body and, with a smile and sense of amusement, mentally let go of any distractive chitter-chatter in your mind. Ask your logic to sit aside and your dreams to come forward.

Step 5

Open your eyes, and imagine yourself 1, 2 or even 3 years from now. Under every heading you created earlier, start to describe what you'd like to create in this area of your life. Let yourself expand and dream. Feel the emotion. Have fun! There is no 'impossible'. There are no limits. Write until you are complete.

Step 6

Bring it all together into one beautiful vision. These questions may assist you, but feel free to make this your own.

What is this extraordinary life like?

_____
_____
_____
_____

Who are you with?

_____
_____
_____
_____

How do you feel in your body?

_____
_____
_____
_____

How do you feel in your mind?

_____

_____

_____

_____

How are you creating income?

_____

_____

_____

_____

What is happening in your business or career?

_____

_____

_____

_____

_____

Clarify Your Vision

What are you doing socially?

How are things with your family?

Are you in love? If so, what does it feel and look like? How are you loving and how are you being loved in return?

Step 7

Finally, what is your 'why'? Why does this vision feel so extraordinary for you? What would the creation of this mean to you? How will it feel?

_____

_____

_____

_____

_____

_____

_____

_____

_____

_____

_____

_____

_____

_____

_____

_____

Step 8

This is your vision! Sit back, absorb it, enjoy it and bring it to life! I will show you how in the next chapter.

Case Study

When Elisa came to see me, she was frustrated with her long-term partner refusing to propose, desperate to start a family and at her wits' end living in a two-room flat while working full time and running a part-time business. She told me she and her partner were tripping over each other's feet, he refused to consider marriage, and as for having a baby? Forget it. She also felt her business was stuck and stagnant as she didn't have the energetic or physical space for it to grow.

I introduced her to this activity, 'Clarify Your Vision'. Elisa embraced it passionately, allowing her subconscious (creative) mind to lead the conversation. Relaxing in one of my lounge chairs, she spoke from her heart. She spoke of the marriage proposal that was on its way and the baby she would have within the next twelve months. She described the house she was going to move into in absolute detail. She envisioned the layout of the rooms, shape and direction of the windows, material of the floor coverings, colour of the walls and its exact physical location.

Within one year Elisa was engaged and pregnant. She had bought the home she had visualised in her mind, and her business was experiencing some well-deserved growth.

Extraordinary!

Bring Your Vision to Life

'I am not engaging in all this self-love and self-growth work to sit on my arse and not build my dream.'

– Stephanie, Extraordinary Client

*M*anifesting. It took me a considerable amount of time to wrap my head around this word. I suspect this is due to so many books, movies and 'gurus' sprouting the belief that if we purely focus on a pretty picture of *anything we want*, it will miraculously appear before us. I wasn't buying it. But the kicker, the hilarious thing, is that I am actually a master at manifesting. I have been creating my world my entire life from the inside out. But, like most humans on the planet, I had no idea I was doing so. I now understand we are creating *all the time*, either consciously or unconsciously.

When I was in my twenties, I had a full-time office job with quite a large corporation. A favourite activity of mine, during bouts of procrastination, was to stare out the window by my desk and dream of a job that would allow me to work outdoors. I also enjoyed turning to the back of my A4 desk diary (no electronic calendars back then) and drooling over the map of the world that was hidden there. I'd grab my highlighter pens and highlight, then re-highlight, all the countries I wanted to visit. I had no idea how I was going to do either of these things. Both seemed to be utterly impossible. They were merely dreams.

One day, out of the blue, a friend called to invite me to join her on some overseas travel she was embarking on the following year. It was a no-brainer! I excitedly began planning my adventure and unexcitedly saving money.

Fast forward to two years later; I'd visited most of the countries depicted in the back of that desk diary and landed a role as road crew for a tour company that spanned Europe, some of Northern Africa, Scandinavia and Russia. Extraordinary travel opportunities while working outside, just as I'd dreamt. It wasn't 'luck' or coincidence; it was synchronicity and creation. I'd taken a dream from my subconscious mind and manifested it, without even realising I was doing it. *Unconscious creation.*

In my thirties, I returned to Australia and recommenced some tertiary education I'd begun prior to my overseas adventure. Towards the completion of my degree, I became aware that an organisation I was interested in working for was about to advertise a role I desperately wanted. This next potential dream job became my primary focus. I studied the organisation's website every day and visualised walking into the building every morning. I polished my resume and purchased a new outfit for the interview. The role was finally advertised, I applied, made it through three (or was it four?) gruelling interviews and was offered the position. I'd had no idea if I was qualified and I'd never worked in that particular industry. Hey, let's be honest, I hadn't had a *'real'* job in over five years! *Unconscious creation.*

This was followed by another dream role, then another after that. All 'unconsciously' created. But, wait, there's more. Let's talk about love.

Decades ago now, I participated in a visualisation activity which involved conceptually entering my 'perfect life', taking note of who and what I was shown to exist there; then returning to my actual life to paint what I'd been given a glimpse of. While I am not very artistic (a three-year-old would have done a better painting), I did my best and set to work recreating what I had seen and experienced. The areas in my life represented in the painting were family and friends, career, love of animals, nature, travel, health and wellbeing. Single at the time, but with dreams of experiencing a loving and healthy relationship, I was overjoyed to have 'seen' myself walking along a red carpet arm-in-arm with a dark-haired man I was clearly about to marry (the wedding dress I was wearing being a huge clue). We were facing away from the observer with only our back profiles in view. Two children walked beside us – a male with dark hair and a female with light coloured hair, matching my own. I assumed the children represented the biological children we would have – the children I would give birth to.

The activity was interesting and fun, and when the paint was dry, I rolled up my painting and took it home. I had no idea if or how that vision would ever physically appear. I was terrible at relationships, consistently chose the 'wrong' men and, as a result, perpetually moved through life in one of two states – single or heartbroken. Initially, I displayed the picture in the inside door of my wardrobe, glancing at it multiple times per day as I rushed around getting dressed for various commitments.

Twelve months later I moved apartments, and it disappoints me that I haven't seen the painting since. It clearly became a casualty of a decluttering cull. Approximately one decade later … *drum roll please* … adorned in a beautiful gown and holding my soulmate's hand, I glided along a red carpet to be married. Our children, biologically his from a previous marriage, walked beside us. Our son has dark hair, like his father, and our daughter's hair is light coloured like her mother's, but also very similar to my own. *Unconsciously created.*

These are easily the most significant and impactful creations I've manifested in my life, *before I realised I was the creator*, before I understood my power. But there have been hundreds, if not thousands more during my fifty years on earth, and not all of them joyful … all while believing, to my core, this 'manifesting' thing was a load of bollocks. My understanding of how the world works, and how we fit into to, is much deeper and clearer now.

Recently, I manifested Handsome Hubby a new car. He told me the make, model, year, colour and price he wanted. For added complexity this car is no longer manufactured, so I was unable to short-cut the process by popping into a dealership and ordering one from the assembly line. The perfect car appeared within two months from the start of the process. To be clear, I did not paste a pretty picture on a vision board and, *bam,* his new car cruised up our driveway. There is more delightful complexity to creation than that.

Bringing your beautiful, extraordinary vision to life takes clarity, belief, faith, patience and *action*. There is no magic wand – you actually have to do some of the work. I have my own daily, weekly and monthly rituals and processes that unlock my action steps – you now have the opportunity to create yours.

If you followed along and completed the activity from Chapter One, you now have a beautiful vision in place. Your vision is crystal clear. It feels right. It feels aligned with your values. You are called to it so powerfully that you cannot help but step into it. You know at a deeply fundamental level that you are here on this planet to do this – it's part of you and the pull towards it is magnetic.

Remember, *everything* you have in your life right now was once an idea, a thought or a vision and *you* brought it to life – consciously or unconsciously. Every resource on the planet is available to you. Every skill, strength and gift you have within you is waiting for your call. Everything you need to bring your vision to life is right here, right now. All that is required is one step.

ACTIVITY

Step 1

Create your ritual of how you will remind yourself of your vision daily.

Personally, I like to write out my vision every single morning. If I have buckets of time, I dive into every gorgeous tiny detail, allowing pages and pages adorned with my loopy handwriting to fall to the floor as I continue to dream, imagine and ultimately create – because that IS what I am doing in that moment. Alternatively, if I have commitments that morning and time is of the essence, I default to the shorter version of this process. Whichever I choose, the end result will always be a vibration of energy as feelings of gratitude overwhelms me – gratitude for the life I currently live, and the one I am currently creating.

If you are more visual, you may prefer an electronic or traditional (pictures and glue) Vision Board. I also love musical reminders. I play motivational songs or YouTube clips that inspire me – anything that reminds me of my power to create.

Jogging is a favourite activity of mine and if you happen to pass me on the footpath you'll hear some fabulously uplifting beats booming from my headphones, or my own voice repeating the mantras of my desires.

We are always creating. We may as well do it consciously. Try them out, have a play, then create your very own daily Vision Reminder Ritual.

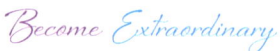

My Vision Reminder Ritual

Bring Your Vision to Life

Tap into your intuition by immediately asking yourself these questions following your daily Vision Reminder Ritual. *What do I feel inspired to do today? What action can I take today to bring this vision closer to me? How will I step in?*

Devise some actions and *do them*. As you move forward, watch the opportunities, people, events, situations, invitations and 'coincidences' appear to assist you in your quest, as if by magic!

_____

_____

_____

_____

_____

_____

_____

_____

_____

_____

_____

Step 3

Move through your day as if you are already living your vision. By becoming the person who is already living this life, and moving into alignment of who that person is, you will naturally begin to think, feel and behave differently. Take the actions they would take and watch your vision begin to take shape!

Step 4

Repeat tomorrow.

Case Study

I met Susie overseas in 2018, and within months she had enrolled as my client. In our first call Susie shared her inspirational vision: a non-for-profit service that would change the face of healthcare. Her vision was so significant, bold and essential it had become too huge (in her mind), rendering her trapped in overwhelm and confusion. Overloaded with information, ideas and possibilities, she did not know where to start. The road ahead of her seemed so long, the thought of travelling the distance drained her of energy. Paralysed by overwhelm, she stopped and did nothing. She was stuck.

Her vision was crystal clear; she could feel it in every cell of her body. She knew exactly what she wanted to create and the positive impact it would have on the community. We needed it to appear.

I asked her what she had tried in the past to bring this vision to life. She told me about her 10-Step Plan. Uh oh. She was very hesitant, but after some persuasion, I convinced her to trial throwing the Plan away. Just for one fortnight. For two weeks only she would trial reminding herself of her vision, tapping into her intuition and then taking the very next step daily. She agreed – as a trial only. She was, as most of us are, very attached to her Plan.

When we jumped into our next call one fortnight later, she was beyond excited! She had taken her first step and guess what happened? Something materialised that wasn't part of her plan until Step 8! In one day she was able to discard Steps 2 to 7!

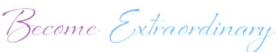

Her project has now launched. She has become the person she wanted to be to create her dream. She sets her actions every day and moves through them (even when she doesn't feel ready). She is transforming herself and creating her vision in the process.

Extraordinary!

Unwrap Your Gifts

'I am now embarking on a new career I thought was too late to pursue.'

– Peter, Extraordinary Client

When I reflect over my life I can see I've spent most of it leaping into situations some would say I had absolutely no business being in. The list is extensive, but the following are the ones that come to mind most readily:

- Moving from a tiny town of 1,200 people to arguably Australia's busiest tourist destination and accepting a finance administration role within a huge international corporation. The job I originally applied for? Waitress.
- Becoming an on-road cook for a European travel company with very little cooking experience. My culinary speciality was 'stuff on toast'.
- Marrying my husband in my mid-forties and becoming an instant stepmother to an 8 and 10-year-old.
- Stepping into my first leadership role.
- Quitting my full time, secure, professional role to create Sky High Coaching.

I embraced every one of these situations with the full understanding that I had *absolutely no idea* what I was doing. Believe me when I say Impostor Syndrome and Fraud Complex are close personal friends of mine (more about them later)! What on Earth possessed me to jump into these situations, ones I knew nothing about and had zero experience in, when failure was a real possibility? It's because I wanted the experience; of exploring my country and the world, making new friends, challenging myself professionally and falling deeply in love.

With non-success definitely possible, how did I ensure the risk was low? How did I back myself? By getting resourceful: utilising the skills I already possessed, unwrapping some gifts I didn't know I had, aligning myself with experts and generous souls who agreed to assist me, reading books, enrolling in courses (and completing them), and working with coaches and mentors.

As mentioned earlier, your birth on this physical plane was no accident. You are supposed to be here, and you arrived carrying a virtual suitcase filled with talents that are unique to you. You have inherent abilities that mean some tasks come to you so easily, you can't understand why other people struggle to perform them. They are more than an action; they are a way of being. For you, they are effortless, and you employ them with minimal conscious thought.

There is no one on the planet like you. No one with your upbringing, parents, siblings, friends, teachers, boyfriends, girlfriends, experiences, coaches, colleagues, bosses, children … you get the picture. The point is there is no one else on Earth identical to you. Comparing yourself to someone else (whether or not you fall short of them or feel superior to them) is of no value. We are incomparable. So let's agree to stop comparing ourselves to others, right here, right now.

You are more resourceful than you realise. Throughout your life you've unwrapped your unique gifts, and developed the skills and strengths required to move through situations and challenges as they arose. In other words, you've used them all to create the world you are experiencing *right now*. And I have some excellent news for you – you haven't unleashed *all* your offerings. In fact, you haven't even come anywhere *close* to doing so.

If your vision is feeling a little daunting right now, if it's feeling so overwhelming that it seems impossible, take comfort and strength in the knowledge that *you* have not completed your evolution. There is still your innate genius to shine and skills to emerge that will support you in your quest. I consider us 'human-evolvings' (just 'being' doesn't appeal to me) and we *only* stop evolving if we choose to. But that's not you, right? So grab the box, tear off the paper, open the lid and see what's inside.

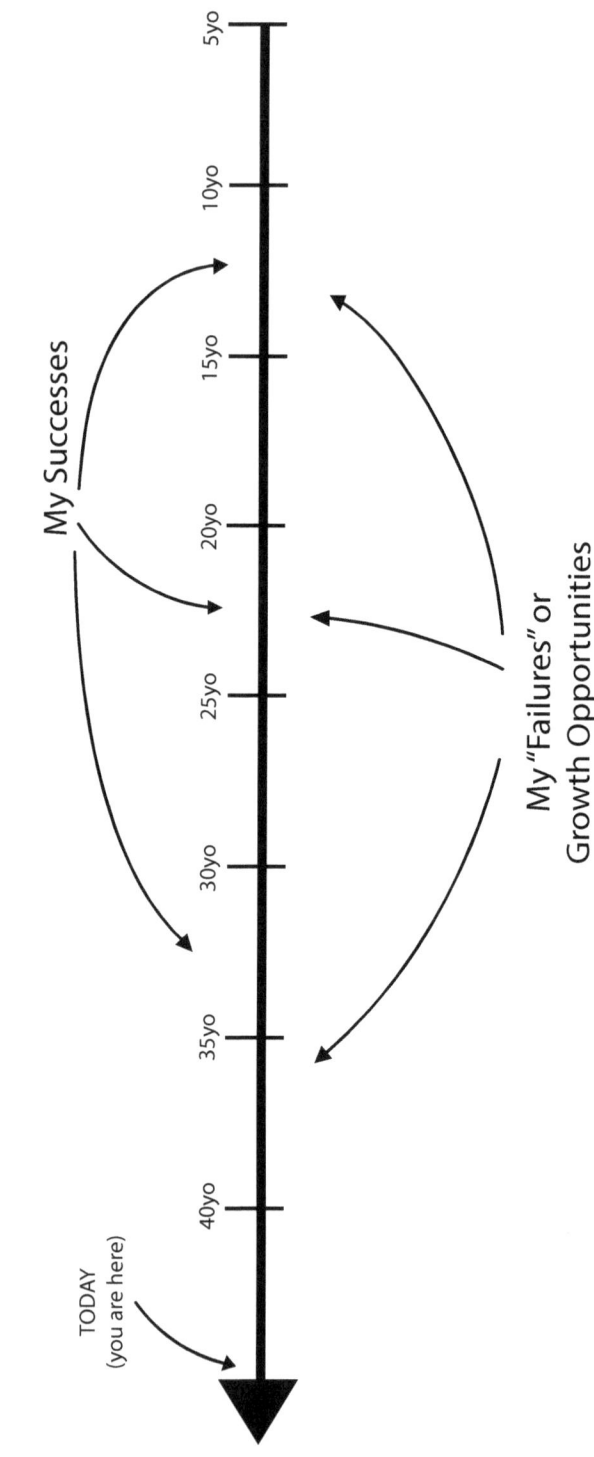

ACTIVITY

Step 1

Create a timeline for your life. List your most successful events and achievements and reflect on how you celebrated them. Now identify all the gifts, skills and strengths you used to create these successful events, projects and milestones.

Step 2

Identify your 'failures' or those projects or dreams that didn't come to fruition – when you've gone belly-up, fallen flat on your face, taken a tumble. Now list all the gifts, skills and strengths that emerged to help move you through these challenging situations.

Step 3

Consider your vision. Circle or highlight every attribute on these two lists you can use today to assist you in the creation your vision, or list them below. These are your Primary Skills (those you've already developed) and Primary Gifts (those you have already unwrapped).

Primary Skills   **Primary Gifts**

_____

_____

_____

_____

_____

_____

_____

_____

_____

_____

_____

_____

Step 4

Are there any skills you can see that, if obtained and/or developed, would assist you in the creation of your vision? If so, let's call these your Secondary Skills. List those and take action towards acquiring or developing them. The action could be reading a book, taking a course, undertaking a qualification, hiring a coach or finding a mentor. Now acknowledge that your Secondary Gifts are those that have not been unwrapped yet, but will come to the fore as you move into your vision. This is *extremely exciting!* Be ready.

Case Study

Paul was referred to me via a previous client. He had recently been made redundant and his unemployment status was spiralling him into despair, negativity and hopelessness. Like most of us when we unexpectedly find ourselves without a job, his professional confidence had taken a beating and his self-doubt had arisen with an almighty force. Personally, he was newly married, his wife had returned to study, and they were living with his parents while renting out their home.

By our second call it was obvious that Paul was not enthused about stepping back into a similar role as before. However, due to his personal situation he naturally felt pressure to take the faster, easier option of jumping back into what he knew, rather than explore exactly what his heart wanted.

Eventually, Paul shared with me his childhood dream of becoming a fireman, a dream he had long left behind due to being, in his mind, far too old. As if he knew I would challenge him in this area, he quickly followed up his admission with the statement that he 'wouldn't pass all the application tests anyway'.

I asked if he would consider allowing the firefighter recruiters to decide if he was too old or not. Could we start looking into all those beautiful and helpful skills, strengths and gifts he'd been hiding away that may assist him in realising his dream? And maybe even uncover some new ones? A huge smile light up his entire face. Whew! Now that we knew what he really wanted to do, we could get to work with some energy and enthusiasm!

Five months later, Paul was accepted into the Fire Brigade Training Program. He graduated three months later and was nominated to be the keynote speaker, on behalf of the graduates, at the graduation ceremony.
Extraordinary!

Smash Through Self-Doubt

'My ability to move through self-doubt has led to me making a positive career change I was too afraid to in the past.'

– Katie, Extraordinary Client

Self-doubt is a colossal subject and often the most significant block to achieving your vision. If you master your self-doubt, you will become a master of your mind and life. Why do we experience self-doubt, where does it come from and how do we smash through it?

It's something I've dealt with a lot myself. In my early thirties, I contacted my personal coach for some coaching. A fixed role I held in my professional life was coming to an end, and I wanted my next step to propel me into a leadership position. Our work together did not disappoint, and within a few months I was appointed into yet another dream role.

A few weeks into this role, I sat with my coach for one of our final meetings. Clasping the herbal tea she kindly provided, I shared with her my enjoyment of my new position and that it was *mostly* going well – except for one small problem. I explained that part of my, and my team's responsibilities, was to encourage our colleagues and members (in the thousands) to participate in a range of health and fitness events such as charitable fun runs. My dilemma, I explained, was that I felt that my team and I should be leading this from the front. We should be entering the events ourselves as inspiration for others.

She observed me curiously and asked why this was a problem, as I was quite fit due to a love of participatory sport and a gym membership. I told her I didn't run.

Without batting an eyelid, she wondered aloud, 'Why not?'

My next words? 'I can't.'

Ah, those voices of self-doubt. The ones that rise up to inform us that we are not:

- Fit enough to complete a fun run
- Lovable enough to attract our soulmate
- Smart enough to start our own business
- Experienced enough to receive the promotion
- Funny enough to be likeable
- Thin or muscly enough to be attractive
- Motivated enough to undertake higher education

Your inner-doubter, your inner critic, can dress it up in as many fancy words as it likes, but the core message is always that *'you are not enough'* – that you are a fraud or an imposter who is not good enough nor worthy enough to be, do or have something you desire. Our inner critic's primary role is to create the appropriate level of doubt and fear within you to prevent you from moving into a situation that may physically or psychologically harm you (*you are 'safe' right where you are, thank you very much!*). Unless addressed and challenged, its success rate can be quite high.

You were not born with any self-doubt. You were born knowing you were limitless, worthy and enough. You came into the world with an understanding of your value, worth and right to experience anything you choose. You only learnt self-doubt after you arrived – via messages from people you trusted and/or direct experiences you've encountered during the course of your life. Have you ever been told *'you are exactly like your mum or dad'*?

Sorry if this is disappointing news for you – but you *are* a product of your parents and other influential adults who contributed to your development during your childhood. I'm sure you've heard the phrase 'children are like sponges' due to their ability to seemingly absorb huge amounts of information at a rapid rate. It is true – they do, and you and I were exactly the same. We are designed that way.

For the first six to ten years of our life, we downloaded everything we saw, heard, or overheard as truth and fact. During your infancy, early and middle childhood, you not only received information via communication from those you trusted, you also moved in and out of life experiences.

Experiences help us give meaning to the world but unfortunately, at a young age, you didn't have a whole lot of life experience to compare it to. If you skipped off to your swimming lesson at age four and it went awry (maybe you had your eyes closed, misjudged the edge of the pool and bonked your head), you may have decided *swimming is bad*. You didn't have the fully-developed brain or the life experience to consider this as nothing more than an unfortunate accident, one that may never be repeated. This may have resulted in you downloading a belief that *swimming is bad*.

We didn't question whether these messages were aligned with our dreams, goals, or who we wanted to be in the world – we weren't equipped to do that. We took the information and downloaded it into our subconscious mind, where it lies fairly dormant as mere information, or morphs into a deeply rooted belief.

So whose thoughts, ideas and beliefs are you actually moving through life with? Your parents'? I invite you to expand your thinking a little more. These thoughts and beliefs most likely didn't begin with your parents – they are just carrying around *their* parents' beliefs! How far back do your beliefs go? It's mind-boggling.

In my case, let's return to my conversation with my coach, regarding my belief of an inability to run. During this stage of my life, I had zero concept of beliefs, helpful or otherwise, so it was my excellent coach who uncovered something I had no idea was residing in my subconscious mind.

As a young child, I suffered childhood asthma and was repeatedly cautioned by adults I trusted (parents, school teachers, sports coaches) that if I was running and felt out of breath, I had to stop. Great advice that served me at the time! I also experienced asthmatic episodes that supported the message I was receiving. Message + Experience = Deeply Ingrained Belief.

By my teenage years, I was no longer being told to stop running if I felt out of breath – I was now the one communicating the message to new physical education teachers and sport coaches. I'd also morphed the message into *'I can't run long distances as I have asthma.'* This worked well for me and I enjoyed being excused from any school running event longer than a few hundred metres ... until one day a new physical education teacher enforced a compulsory 1500m run – no exceptions. Halfway through the event, I withdrew, gasping for breath. This is the final time I can recall having an asthmatic episode.

Fast forward to adulthood. I told myself (and anyone else I had to, such as personal trainers) that I did not run because I Could Not. Definite. Full stop. Capital letters. Almost daring someone to challenge me.

The belief was intense and deeply ingrained, but it was not unhelpful. I played netball, swam, walked, went to the gym. It was not preventing me from doing anything I loved in any way ... that is until I found myself in my new leadership role, with a desire to lead and inspire others to participate in fun runs!

Once my coach and I could see this clearly, we worked through the exact activity I have shared with you in this chapter. We identified the unhelpful belief (*I can't run*), we found the source (messages received from people I trusted, and experiences that supported those messages – the double whammy). We recognised it was false (I had outgrown my childhood asthma), we created a new, simple belief (*I can run*) and I started creating evidence to prove its truth and download it into my subconscious mind. I began by running one block, then walking one block, and built from there. I now love fun runs, and my longest distance achieved is a half marathon.

Our Subconscious Mind

You can see how those beliefs I had at the back of my mind were hindering me. A belief is just a belief that sits quietly in your subconscious mind until it's called upon or triggered. 'Okay,' you may be thinking. 'So what? What's all the fuss about?' The fuss is that your subconscious mind is the part of your brain that's 'flying your plane'. You think your conscious mind is? Think again.

Your conscious mind (also known as the objective mind) can think, reason, analyse, make plans for the future, solve problems, learn, compare and identify incoming information from your external environment via your senses. It processes external stimuli at .40 per second.[1]

Meanwhile, your subconscious mind handles all the functions you don't ever think about, such as breathing, regulating our body temperature and cell regeneration. When you sleep, your conscious mind rests, but your subconscious mind does not. It is also a huge storage area (think of a USB) where your store your beliefs and your programs.

---
1. *The Biology of Belief,* Bruce H. Lipton, Ph.D

Part of its role is to ensure you behave according to your beliefs and programs. It is much faster and more powerful than the conscious mind, processing 20,000,000 environment stimuli per second.[2]

Whilst the subconscious mind is our back seat pilot, the conscious mind is our manual control. When I recently found myself, whilst driving, in the pathway of car which had run a red light, it was my subconscious mind that caused my foot to slam on the brake.

My conscious mind, which responds to external stimuli at a much slower rate, did not have time to be aware of the impending threat. Your subconscious mind scans your environment for cues or 'triggers' and immediately employs previously learned behaviours – all without any assistance or awareness of the conscious mind.

My subconscious mind came to the rescue – the only part of me that is able to process external stimuli, and react, at that speed. The previously learned behaviour was how to drive a car (foot on brake makes car stop) which was undertaken by my conscious mind.

Do you remember when you learned to drive? It seemed so confusing and challenging and you spent most of the time 'in your head' trying to coordinate all the actions required – it almost seemed impossible to watch the road, and every other vehicle using it, at the same time!

Once you downloaded 'how to drive a car' into your subconscious mind, where all programs are stored and appear when needed, you can drive whilst simultaneously thinking about your family or your career or what's for dinner tonight. If you are a driver, and have been for a while, I'm sure you've experienced arriving at your destination and feeling a little panicked that you don't remember the actual journey.

Don't worry. You didn't run a red light, hit a parked car or leave a trail of damage in your wake. Your subconscious mind guided you very safely to your destination. Together your

---

2. Same as above.

two levels of mind are a dynamic duo! But all superpowers can be used for good *or* evil! They can serve us, or hinder us.

Negative Self-Talk

Have you ever wanted something so badly you could taste it? You made plans and put the wheels in motion. You tried so hard and are so sure you did all the 'right' things, but it didn't eventuate?

It's so confusing, you have no idea what went wrong, or why it hasn't appeared. Is everyone else just luckier or smarter or more motivated than you? No, they are not. You may be harbouring an unhelpful belief that is sabotaging your dreams.

How do you know? By watching your language – the messages you tell yourself, as well as others. If you allow your Inner Critic to take control, you may find yourself a victim of Impostor Syndrome or Fraud Complex (*I am not good enough to be here*); Self-Doubt (*I can't do this*) and Self-Sabotage (unconscious thought patterns and behaviours that hold you back).

Are you familiar with the 'voice' of your inner critic? It's the thought that flies in to inform you you're not motivated enough get fit, not desirable enough to find love, not smart enough to manage your finances, not experienced enough to be promoted or not talented enough to grow your business... *insert your own voice here*. If you listen to the voice, and repeat its message to yourself and others, you are strengthening the belief it is attached to. Having a thought is *not* thinking. It's time to get curious about your thoughts.

Warning! If your belief was downloaded at a young age and deeply ingrained, this may not be an easy task. Find a professional to assist you. It will be worth it.

ACTIVITY

Step 1

To identify if you are harbouring an unhelpful belief, reflect on your language. Unhelpful beliefs usually start with one of the following:

I can't …
I don't …
I won't …
I'm not …
I am …

Generalising may also identify an unhelpful belief, such as 'all politicians are corrupt'. This is a very definitive language that leaves no room for growth or expansion of the mind. It's closed thinking.

Step 2

If you can pinpoint how and when you downloaded the belief, it may be helpful to identify how it could have served you once, but is now no longer relevant or required. If you can't recall, that is okay. Just move on to the third step.

_____

_____

_____

_____

_____

Step 3

In this step, we recognise that the belief is false. You have downloaded this belief in the past, and you are not that person anymore (even if you were yesterday). You have evolved, developed and grown since then. Make a conscious choice to release it.

Step 4

You have identified your unhelpful belief and recognised that it's untrue! Nice work! What new, empowering belief would you love to wake up to everyday instead? What would you like to believe instead? Write it down (even if you don't believe it yet)!

_____

_____

_____

_____

_____

_____

_____

Step 5

Start downloading your new, empowering belief right now! Allocate some time – at least an hour – and reflect over your entire life.

Draw out examples that align with this new belief. Begin collecting evidence of actions you've taken that align with your new, empowering belief.

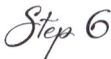
Step 6

Step into your new belief every single day. This is the ongoing work that takes dedication, commitment and a desire to leave the past behind and live in the present. Remind yourself of your new belief every morning before you leave home – in writing or song or picture, however it works best for you. Choose to lean into that belief and move into your day with that intention. Live it!

Take daily actions that align with the belief, which may feel uncomfortable at first, then record them by writing them down. Some clients choose to record their new actions in the moment (notes on phone or small notebook), while others prefer to record them at the end of the day.

If you remain committed to your new belief, celebrate new choices, new actions, and collect evidence of support, your new belief will form and become automatic.

_____

_____

_____

_____

_____

Case Study

Lynn is an old friend who contacted me when she heard I'd become a personal coach. A vice-principal in the private school system, she had spent the previous year applying for principal roles without success.

The most frustrating part of the process, she confided, was that she continually 'finished second' in the recruitment process. I felt her disgruntlement – how annoying to be constantly placed second. She had been a vice-principal for many years, knew she had the experience and the qualifications for the top job – she just didn't know what she was doing wrong.

Very early into our work together, Lynn brought forth a memory she thought she'd forgotten. During one of her senior years in secondary school, a teacher had repeatedly informed her that when it came to her career she would make a fantastic second-in-command – that she would achieve a certain amount of success no matter whatever industry she chose, but she would never achieve a position at the highest level.

Lynn had downloaded the belief that she was only worthy enough to be 'second-in-command' or second when it came to her career. Lying quietly in her subconscious mind, this powerful belief came running when she stepped into an interview for a principal position. Even though her conscious mind desired the role, her belief was more powerful. It created an element of doubt whether she was worthy enough for the appointment and unbeknownst to her, that doubt was visible to interview panels she presented herself to.

> *The metaphorical lightbulb switched on – Lynn could see her situation clearly and took the action required to delete this belief.*
>
> *Some short weeks later she applied for another principal role, and was appointed into the position without hesitation.*
>
> *Extraordinary!*

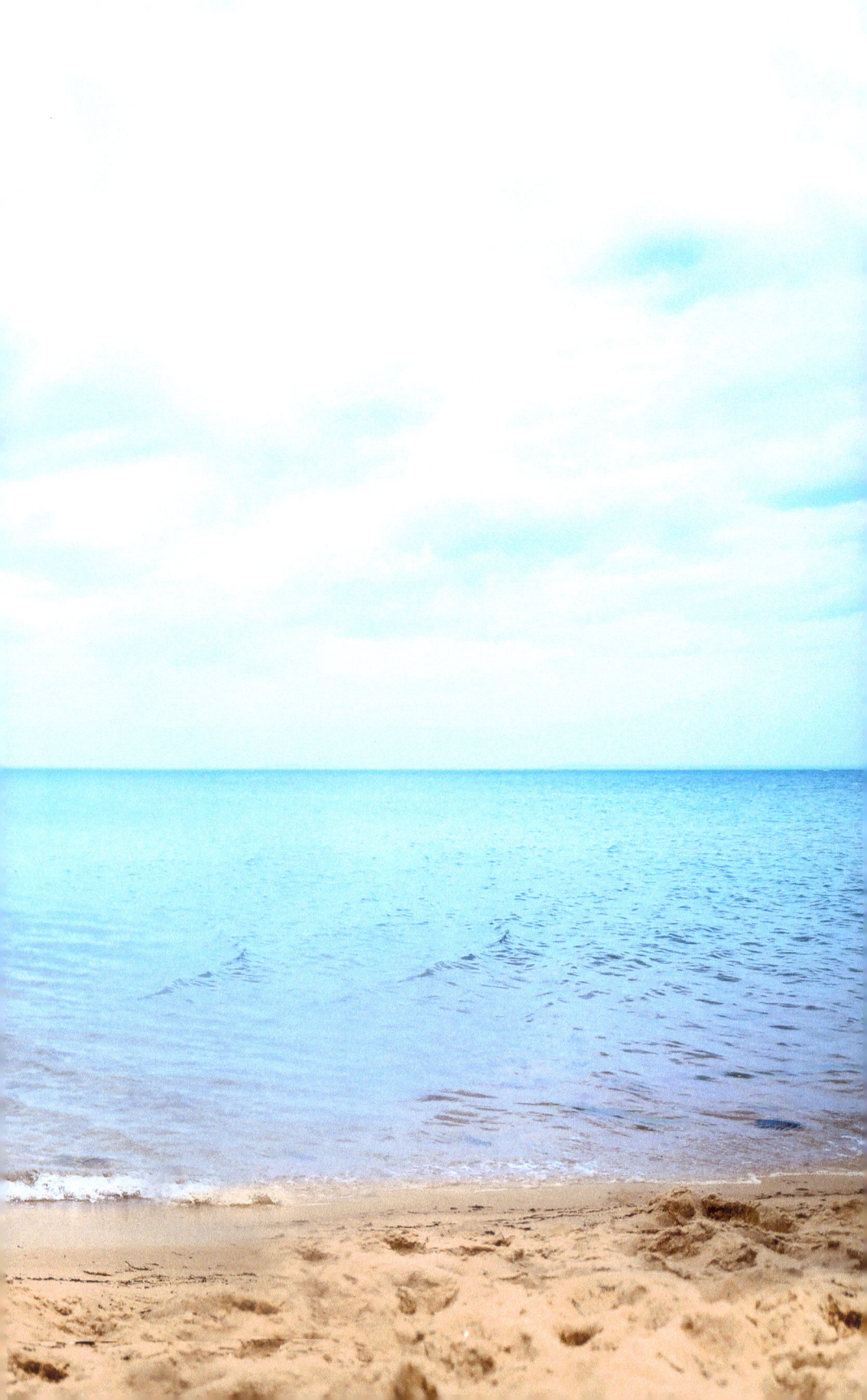

Create More Confidence

'Being able to catch my negative thoughts before they impact my behaviour has changed my life personally and professionally.'

– *Gabrielle, Extraordinary Client*

Have you ever laughed in your boss's face? I have! And all because he had the audacity to *believe in me*, when I didn't believe in myself.

We were in his office for a Monday morning catch up when he asked if I was aware that a recent opening had become available in the upper echelon of our organisation. When I replied that I was, he enquired if I was throwing my hat into the ring. Was I applying for this role? Queue my impromptu, and fairly loud, laughter.

As I wiped the tears from my eyes and regained my composure, I realised his gaze had turned to one of puzzlement. I quickly threw my soggy tissue in the bin and returned his look with one of my own – amazement. Things had suddenly turned very serious. I cleared my throat and admitted that I had not given one thought to applying for this role as I felt it was beyond my abilities. For the next ten minutes or so he conveyed why he thought I was perfect for the role and the value I would bring to that department. As I left his office, promising to consider his suggestion, he told me it was time for me to step into a new challenge, to grow in my career.

I would love to tell you that I put my big girl pants on and applied for the role – that I felt the fear and did it anyway, and learned so much about myself in the process. But, alas, I did not. The woman I was back then did not have the confidence in herself, nor her abilities, to make such a bold move.

What is confidence and why are so many of us craving more of it? How many times have you heard someone say they would have done or created something if only they'd felt more confident? Is there something you would have tried, reached for, attempted, stepped into, agree to ... if only you'd felt a little more confident?

The *Oxford Dictionary* defines 'confident' as:

> *1. Feeling or showing confidence in oneself of one's abilities or qualities.*
>
> *2. Feeling or showing certainty about something.*

Most of my clients over the years have expressed that they would love to feel more confident, but they don't want confidence just for the sake of having confidence. They crave more confidence because they want to experience what having more confidence would bring them. They want to experience a greater feeling of certainty in themselves.

If you have found yourself feeling a little unconfident in any area of your life, then I extend some huge *congratulations* to you. This tells me you are stepping into a larger arena. You are moving out of your familiar zone and into the unknown. When we take a risk, accept a challenge or make ourselves vulnerable, we feel fear. It is a normal part of being human.

Lack of confidence can show up as many guises, such as fear of failure, performance anxiety, self-doubt, procrastination, paralysis by analysis, and the anxiety of imagining the outcome of a new situation and making it unfavourable.

When we feel unconfident it creates quite an uncomfortable feeling in our body, and unlocks the annoying inner critic in our mind. That critic loves to send you messages of failure, unworthiness and how badly you're going to mess this up!

When faced with a situation we feel unconfident in, we search for a way to release the fear and tension within, something to help us *make it through* the event or experience. What do we tend to grab hold of first? Usually we reach for our favourite crutch, the most common example being alcohol or drugs. None readily available, or not really your thing? You may choose to hide your lack of confidence by donning your invisible armour and bulldozing your way through the situation.

Directing the spotlight away from you and towards others is also an effective way to cloak your discomfort and lack of confidence. Popular distraction techniques include making others laugh at your own or someone else's expense, gossiping or speaking negatively about others.

Finally, and easily the most effective technique to hide your lack of confidence, is to not to put yourself in the situation at all! You may do this by avoiding speaking up in meetings, raising your hand to run the new team project, applying for the promotion, going on a date, joining a yoga class, attending the party, launching your business idea or writing the book that's been inside you for years.

You remain in your familiar situation that does not bring you true inner happiness and fulfilment because you do not have the confidence to move into something new – something that has the potential to be extraordinary! The fear of rebuff, rejection or perceived failure is just too high.

What would you do and who would you be if only you had a little more confidence? What new or different choices would you make and what new or different actions would you take? What if life was an endless choice of possibilities, yours for the taking?

Let's return to the definition of confident, because I absolutely *love* how helpful it is to us.

> 1. Feeling or *showing* confidence in oneself of one's abilities or qualities.
> 2. Feeling or *showing* certainty about something.

Boom! You don't have to be feeling the confidence to ooze it! You can show it and be within the definition. Even if your hands are clammy, your tummy is full of butterflies, that red rash has crept up your neck and you think you might lose your lunch all over your new shoes – if you can learn to *show* confidence, regardless of how you're feeling on the inside, you are already there. Unwavering confidence, here we come!

We, as humans, have a misconception that thought leads straight to action. I encourage you to expand your mind. As we learned in the previous chapter, we carry around a plethora of beliefs in our subconscious minds that are triggered by external stimuli. When the belief is triggered, it creates a thought. That thought flies in (seemingly from nowhere), and evokes an emotion. It is that emotion that drives you to take action. This is how we create our world from the inside out. If a thought flies in with the message that you are not good enough, smart enough, qualified enough, fit enough, loveable enough, funny enough, or experienced enough to be, do or have whatever it is you want, your confidence falters.

The message, if given energy and consciousness (in other words, you give it power) creates a response in your body. This is why you experience physical sensations when you feel unconfident about a situation you are about to step into;

nausea, sweaty palms, rashes, butterflies, tension, heaviness, difficulty speaking, faster heart rate, perspiration etc. What if you could stop giving your Inner Critic power, thus disrupting the signal (and therefore unhelpful responses) before it makes it to the body?

Working on your unhelpful beliefs (as outlined in the previous chapter) will absolutely assist with decreasing and/or eliminating these unhelpful thoughts. However, be aware that there is a part of your brain designed to scan for danger (it's how we stay alive).

Perfect storm, right? You're about to step into something different, bigger or brighter than ever before. A part of your brain called the amygdala is scanning for something that could potentially be dangerous and zeros in on this new or unfamiliar situation, then attempts to steer you away from the potentially dangerous situation by sending you a fearful (negative) thought intended to stop you in your tracks. The way our brain is wired results in all of us having a certain amount of negative, or unhelpful, thoughts per day.

Busting Our Unhelpful Thoughts

Have you ever experimented with an exercise that was designed to stop you having unhelpful, or negative, thoughts? I have. The instruction was to wear a rubber band around my wrist all day and whenever a negative thought flew in I was to flick my wrist with the rubber band. While the exercise did make me more aware of my unhelpful thoughts, it certainly did not eliminate them, and I ended up with a lovely red welt on my wrist.

If we can't stop negative or unhelpful thoughts entirely, what do we do instead? We can refuse to give them power when they swoop in. We give them power by giving them consciousness and energy – paying attention to them, believing them or by pushing against them. Let's do the opposite. Let's pull the power plug.

These are some techniques myself, and my clients, have used successfully to decrease or eliminate the power of our negative thoughts.

1. **Send the thoughts away!** Learning to send the thoughts away when they swoop in is one of the most effective techniques, but does take some practise to become automatic. Spend ten minutes in a quiet place, allowing every thought you have (good, bad or ugly) to float in, then (without giving it any energy) wait for it to float out again. Practising this daily will help you cultivate the skill so it will come easily to you in a more stressful real-life situation.

2. **Make friends with your Self Saboteur!** If you have an unhelpful message that frequently arises as if it's on repeat, turn and face it. If a message flying in is unhelpful, undesirable and making you feel 'bad', it is a lie. It is currently a part of you, but it is not the essence of who you are. I can guarantee you weren't born with that voice; it's attached itself to you at some point in your life (return to the previous chapter if required).

    Clients have found it helpful to give the origin of that message a form – for example, a funny name, a face and an identity. Some clients have made friends with their saboteur. Other clients even manage to laugh at their saboteur. The crux of the exercise is understanding the message is not valid – it is not you, but the part of you designed to keep you safe from harm.

3. **Sing!** Next time an unhelpful thought swoops in, sing it. Imitate the voice of a singer who makes you laugh or a singer you love. Pop in some imaginary music. Have a boogie. Anything that diminishes its power.

4. **Silly voice.** Can you take Walt Disney's Donald Duck seriously? Or Sesame Street's Elmo? Give the unhelpful thought a silly voice, one that makes you chuckle.

5. **Use your computer.** This activity has been used very successfully by clients when they are working in an office, surrounded by colleagues. When the unhelpful message swoops in (before the meeting, presentation or interview) type it into a Word document (or similar) and manipulate the words on your screen in various ways. Not only can this make you laugh, it also illustrates thoughts only have the power *you* give them – you are ultimately the one in control.

Which of these techniques do you think would work most effectively for you?

Imagine you're about to walk into that interview, meet that fantastic person for your first date, give your very first presentation, step into a new networking event, send your book manuscript to your editor ... your thoughts are flying in with an urgency and force, screaming at you to stop! Warning you of all the dangers – all the things that could go wrong.

Now imagine letting them float on by, shushing your self-saboteur (with a smile), turning them into an amusing song, morphing them into a humorous voice or making them so tiny and faint you can hardly see them on your computer screen! There's no battle or attachment and you can redirect all your energy and consciousness to the task or event on hand.

And what happens when you are fully engaged (directing all energy and consciousness) into the task or event on hand? You are completely *present* and *focused*. When you are absolutely immersed in the task at hand, or event in play, you can be certain that you are showing up your very best self. You're not worried about the outcome. You're not obsessing over what others may be thinking. You've released any fear.

You are engaged with the panel of interviewers.

You are interested and focused on the person across the table on your date.

You enjoy making eye contact and sharing information with your audience during your presentation.

You relish connecting with others at the networking event.

You congratulate yourself on your dedication and commitment as you send your manuscript to your publisher.

You are cultivating more confidence, right in that moment.

But what if an unhelpful thought catches you unawares, your confidence begins to waiver, and some uncomfortable feelings arise in your body? Don't despair – I've got you!

Remind yourself that, as per the *Oxford Dictionary*'s definition, *showing* confidence (even when you're are not feeling it) is still confidence! Do you think you can *feel* 100% confident in any activity or situation, without any prior practise or experience in that activity or situation? The answer is no. It's impossible.

Taking *action* creates real, rock-solid confidence. If you are waiting to feel more confident before you decide to step into something that's bigger or brighter or bolder than before, you are going to be waiting a very long time.

I invite you to take a moment, and bring forth in your mind something in your life you feel extremely capable and confident in right now. Reflect back a little further. How confident did you feel when you first stepped into this situation, activity or task? When it was new and different? Hopefully, you can see how the actions of confidence come first, and the feelings follow.

Actions of Confidence

How do you generate your *Actions of Confidence* when you are stepping into something completely new; onto a bigger stage or into a more expansive arena? How do we ooze poise and confidence when we may not be particularly feeling it, without the benefit of prior rehearsal or experience?

These are the techniques I myself and my clients use when we wish to show confidence when embarking on a new endeavour:

1. **Prepare, prepare, prepare.** Write down everything you can do to prepare for the event, and take action.

2. **Seek help.** This may be in the form of skills training, personal or professional development (partner with a mentor or coach), reading books or undertaking a course. Is there a friend or family member with some experience in this area you can approach for insight and advice?

3. **Keep your action steps as tiny as you can.** While transformation involves stepping out of our familiar zone, too broad a jump may cause the fear to take over and tip you into 'flight, fright or freeze'.

4. **Live by your values**. Identify your top five values and live in alignment with them. Falling asleep every night knowing you lived in alignment with what's most important to you cultivates confidence in decision making.

5. **List the people who matter**. Make a list of five or fewer people who really matter in your life. Becoming detached from other people's thoughts and feelings about you helps cultivate confidence.

6. **Consider your body language.** Are you aware of what external indicators, such as your posture and facial expressions, say about you? Clients in my confidence workshops have identified the following body language traits are shown by people they perceive as confident: making eye contact, standing up straight, keeping their hands visible (not hiding

them in pockets), keeping their limbs still (fidgeting was seen as a sign of nervousness), having a firm handshake, and most of all, *smiling*.

7. **Project confidence through your voice.** Clients in my confidence workshops have identified the following verbal cues are shown by people they perceive to be confident: articulating a statement as a definite statement, not a question; smiling when they speak (even on the phone), being comfortable with silence and pauses in conversation, using limited 'filler words' such as um and ah, not speaking too fast, and speaking clearly with the correct amount of volume and projection for the situation.

8. **Build your resilience,** which we will be discussing later in this book.

If you use some or all of the tools and techniques outlined in this chapter, the emotional responses that arise in your body when you are feeling a little (or a lot) unconfident should begin to decrease – even disappear entirely.

But what if they don't? What if nausea, sweaty palms, rashes, butterflies, tension, heaviness, difficulty in speaking, faster heart rate and perspiration pop up right before you step into your brand new creation, situation, event or challenge? Let's spin those feelings on their head!

This tactic has been working for me for years, and as I teach it to clients, they tell me it's working for them, too!

I invite you to bring forth the memory of a time you were *extremely* excited about something you were about to experience – your graduation, your first leadership role, your wedding, your first child being born, stepping onto the podium to receive your gold medal, your first book being published ... *insert your own here.* Can you identify the feelings that arise in your body when you are absolutely thrilled?

Attendees of my confidence workshops have agreed that the feelings of *excitement* we experience are the same, or certainly similar, to the feelings of *nervousness*: nausea, sweaty palms, rashes, butterflies, tension, heaviness, difficulty in speaking, faster heart rate and perspiration. As I am regularly challenging myself, repeatedly stepping into arenas I may not have any business being in, frequently feeling the fear … I remind myself these feelings are ones of *excitement, not fear*. They are a signal to move forward, not to stop! This disruption to a habitual thought pattern works successfully for me and my clients. Have a play, give it a try and see what you think.

ACTIVITY

Step 1

Think of something you would do if only you had a little more confidence. Write down what it is, why you'd love to have that experience, and how moving into it would enhance you and/or your life.

_____

_____

_____

_____

_____

Step 2

Close your eyes and imagine you were obligated to take this step right now. Mentally and deeply place yourself in the situation. Notice what happens in your mind and your body. On a scale of one to ten, mark how confident you would be if you had to go out into the world and do this thing *right now*.

1   2   3   4   5   6   7   8   9   10

Step 3

Go back through this chapter, pull out the suggested tools and techniques you think will work for you and have a play with them. Maybe there's a situation you could try them in today?

_____

_____

_____

_____

_____

_____

_____

Step 4

Mark a date on your calendar for two days from now (or however long you decide to experiment with the tools) and revisit your scale. If we sent you out into the world on this day, after you've trialled some new confidence techniques, where does your confidence sit on the scale?

1   2   3   4   5   6   7   8   9   10

Step 5

If it has increased, congratulations. If not, keep practising the techniques, or try some different ones until you move up the scale.

Case Study

Richard came to work with me when he realised he was falling behind in his career. In his early thirties, Richard had grown tired of congratulating peers upon their promotions while he stayed stuck in the same role year after year.

We met in an upmarket hotel lobby and, as he loosened his tie to relax, he disclosed that he knew why he was being overlooked by his superiors. Richard lacked confidence in public speaking and actively avoided delivering presentations. Not ideal (for him), as every leader in the organisation he worked for was required to give regular updates on products and services to staff and clients via on-stage presentations. He knew he was holding himself back in his career, understood change was required, and he wanted it to happen fast. He told me that at the mere suggestion of him being the next person in his team to deliver the monthly product update, his lack of confidence would show itself in the form of unhelpful thoughts and physical symptoms. And not just some of the symptoms outlined in this chapter – all of them! The physical symptoms would become so intense that he would call into work 'sick' on the day of his scheduled presentations. His entire being was not only determined to keep him 'safe' in his familiar zone, it was highly successful.

Richard utilised many of the tools and techniques mentioned in this chapter, but the one that served him most powerfully was stepping forward (raising his hand to deliver a presentation) then preparing for it.

During our work together he stepped into an action he set for himself. He approached his boss and requested an opportunity to present the details of his latest project at the next All Staff Meeting. It was accepted.

Next, Richard embraced the next action he'd set for himself – preparation. To begin, he learned how to send unhelpful thoughts on. Next, he wrote the presentation content and designed the PowerPoint slides. Finally, he practised his delivery – to himself, his children's toys (a personal favourite preparation tool of my own), his family and then to some supportive friends.

By the time the staff meeting rolled around, he could recite his presentation forwards and backwards. He still felt some nerves, but his performance was a success.

In his own words:

> 'Since working with Janelle I have gone from almost no public speaking to giving at least one presentation to small and large groups every week. I can move forward in my career with the knowledge that I have valuable content to share and the confidence that I can present it in a clear and engaging way.'

Extraordinary!

Raise Your Resilience

'I am calmer, stronger and more resilient. The freedom I feel is exhilarating!'

– Sidonie, Extraordinary Client

In 2011 my world as I knew it collapsed. In the space of three months, I suffered a miscarriage (at 12 weeks), my mother passed away from cancer three weeks after diagnosis, and I found the courage to walk away from an unhappy and unhealthy relationship. The following months were, without doubt, the worst of my life. Lost and confused, angry and heartbroken, I found it difficult to function. Life felt dark, confusing, difficult and cruel. Who, I wondered, had switched off the light? And how do I turn it back on?

As I emerged from winter and stepped into spring, the sun poked its head out from behind a cloud and winked. I began to notice the beauty of Mother Nature again, feel the love of friends and family and feel warmth on my face. I realised I could smile, then eventually laugh. Life moves on, I decided, and life is a wonderful adventure.

We all encounter challenging moments, people, situations and we all suffer periods of feeling defeated. We all get knocked down and we all have bruises. Our bruises may appear due to 'normal' life experiences often outside our control, such as the death of a loved one, the breakdown of a relationship, the loss of a job, a business collapsing or a health scare. They may also develop due to conscious steps we choose to take ourselves, such as courageously stepping off our edge, playing a bigger game, trying something new or breaking our mould … and falling flat on our face! Ouch!

I was sacked from my very first part-time job when I was fifteen because I copied the behaviour of one of the older staff members. Apparently, bosses could show inconsistency. Who knew? I was bullied so severely by a boss in my first full-time role it took decades for my fear of the words *'Can I see you in my office for a minute?'* to subside. I was made redundant from a recruitment agency at twenty-one years old.

Decades of equestrian riding and sporting competitions saw me successful but also, at times, defeated. A broken engagement at twenty years old was only the beginning of a string of failed romances, spanning two decades. In my early thirties, I wrote a book that was never published.

In my early forties, I launched Sky High Coaching. If you are an entrepreneur, solopreneur or small business owner, you'll understand when I say that this business caper, this creative process that starts and ends with you, has the power to raise you to dizzying heights … then spin you into a cycle of self-doubt, sometimes in the very same hour.

The day after experiencing a major earthquake whilst facilitating a Sky High Coaching retreat in Bali, I was privy to some very wise words from our host. She told me, *'The world is supposed to be in chaos. It's we who try to put in it order'*. Natural phenomena such as volcanic eruptions, hurricanes, earthquakes, superstorms, bushfires, floods and drought are part of the earth's evolution. We attempt to eliminate the perceived chaos because we fear a loss of control. If we can keep control, we are safe from harm. That is the basic premise. If we can predict what's going to happen, when it's going to happy and how it's going to happen, we can plan and prepare. We can build our fort, don our armour, raise our sword and we will be safe.

This is the myth, or misconception, of what some people consider resilience to be. *'I am going to armour-up and smash my way through life. Nothing can stop me! Nothing can hurt me!'* They believe the foundation of resilience is survival and the avoidance of risk.

For me, that is not what true resilience is. True resilience is the freedom to be who we are and live how we wish to live – to be courageous enough to display our vulnerabilities, take chances and risk messing up! True resilience is not donning your armour and raising your sword, intent on protecting yourself from pain and disappointment. It's moving through life with the freedom to love and trust whilst understanding, at the deepest level, that you will always be *okay* no matter what happens around you. True resilience is the profound inner certainty that your roots are strong, you are infinitely loved and supported and your vision is clear. You are living aligned with your values and when the proverbial hits the fan (because it does and it will), *you can, and will, handle it.*

There's a great saying, *'God looks at our plans and laughs'.* There's another excellent saying, *'Bad things don't happen to good people. Bad things happen to all people.'* It's part of your physical experience on Earth. You will experience setbacks as you move through life. You will experience failure. Obstacles will appear. You will procrastinate. There will be days when it all seems too hard and overwhelming, and it will feel more natural to stay in your comfort zone. There will be times that no matter how well defined your plans are, they just won't unfold as you would have liked.

- Printers crash when the report is due
- Amazing employees resign
- Unrequired love is real
- Injuries are sustained eight weeks before the event

- Home renovations begin years after their intended date
- Unexpected bills arrive
- The promotion goes to someone else
- Projects run late
- Someone leaves
- Someone is unkind
- Accidents happen
- Mother Nature does her thing

We can choose to stay stuck. We can choose to fall into victim-status and collapse into blame of others, ourselves or life! Or we can choose to reframe challenges, open our minds and expand and grow – to flourish from setbacks, rather than allow them to set us back; to consider if we have been protected and/or redirected.

Sometimes the most unexpected disappointments show themselves, in time, to be the greatest of gifts. We are such a resilient species; we literally have the capacity to grow even when our hearts are breaking. Suffering is all around us, but so are beautiful things. Terrible tragedies also bring tremendous growth and strength.

Ever met one of those people who seems to be eternally happy all the time – and I don't mean faking it; I mean they are authentically joyful and energetic? That's a choice they make. Their life isn't charmed. They have hardships just like everyone else. They choose to live their life with resilience.

The good news is we were born with a certain amount of resilience. If we'd given up the moment we fell, we'd still be crawling around on our hands and knees. The great news is we can raise our resilience to a more extraordinary level, and we don't have to wait until a tragic event hits us to do so. Begin to practice these following techniques and feel your resilience rise!

Positivity

Life loves throwing us little unexpected surprises. Technology will fail. People will change their minds. You fall ill the day of the huge presentation. Weather will impede events or training. You'll get stuck in traffic at the worst possible time.

When a challenge arises, acknowledge the bad, but seek out the good. Practice saying things like, '*Yes, the system may have crashed, but I'm so happy the membership database remained intact.*'

Live to Learn

As the famous saying goes, sometimes you win, and sometimes you learn. When a challenge arises, look for the opportunity to grow and evolve. Seek a solution, rather than obsessing over the problem. Get curious about what this situation may be able to teach you.

Open Your Heart

When we practise acts of kindness and serve others, it creates a feeling of wellbeing inside us. When we feel well, we feel secure, happy and healthy, and thus more resilient.

Practise Gratitude

What are you grateful for when it comes to your personal and professional life? There are many ways to remind yourself what you are thankful for each day – a vision board, a journal, a daily email to a friend or a daily appreciation ritual.

Physical and Emotional Health

Whilst physical and emotional health is important to all of us, it's something to pay particular attention to if you are focusing on bringing an extraordinary vision to life.

The last thing you want is to fall ill. Create a daily routine that includes a good night's sleep, excellent nutrition, some exercise, and being still.

When we are still or 'doing nothing', our brain uses the time to process data and file it away – in other words, it cleans up! How fantastic! You can be still in a structured way such as meditation, but it will work just as well chilling in the backyard.

Humour

Laughing in the face of adversity is healing for your mind and body. This can be a toughie at times, but if you can manage it, you'll reap the benefits.

Flexibility and Adaptability

Unless you are very lucky or very savvy, when you start moving towards something new or different, you don't know what you don't know.

Businesses change and fluctuate as they grow. Sportspeople suffer injuries they did not anticipate. Those on a quest for love find themselves in the position of both rejecter and rejectee. You realise the new incredible role you landed was actually the wrong move for you. Things will go awry.

Be ready to roll with the changes. Remember to learn, grow and evolve, too.

Optimism

The most successful people are those who are optimistic about the future. They keep going because they are certain it will all work out in the end. They understand setbacks are just temporary, and obstacles are learning opportunities.

Decisiveness

As human-evolvings, feeling 'stuck' makes us feel very uncomfortable because we are designed to continually move forward. Making clear and strong decisions helps us feel more confident and in control. If you realise a decision you made was the 'wrong' one, learn from it and change course.

Know Your Values

We all have the most amazing internal compass inside us, and that is guided by 'your values'. Sit down and work out what your top five values are today. What is most important to you right now? Knowing your values, and living aligned with them, increases confidence in decision making. If you are always honouring your values, it is a little harder for life's challenges to knock you off course.

Breathe!

You realise the report you've procrastinated over is due in an hour. If you don't hand this in on time your boss will not be happy and it may jeopardise your upcoming promotion.

Feeling the pressure, you put your head down, butt up and bang out some mediocre work. You feel disappointed in your efforts but send it to print and race to the machine. From one metre away, you can see the red light blinking. Someone has jammed the machine and walked away. You see red!

When small glitches happen in seemingly rapid succession, it has the power to bring the entire day down on top of us. We can yell or stamp our feet, or we can take two minutes to stop and breathe.

Any yogi will tell you the power of breath is underestimated. Move away from the situation (even five steps will help) and take some deep breaths in and out. You will be amazed by how much more resilient you'll feel in just a few minutes.

Develop Your Communication Skills

It is highly likely that you will need to communicate with others as you move towards your vision. Other people can work with you or against you, affecting your resilience. Hone your written, verbal and non-verbal communication skills to a level where you can communicate your needs, while nurturing and appreciating personal and professional relationships.

Call on Your Support System

Creating a professional or personal vision can be the loneliest quest in the world. When things are tough, it's easy to feel isolated and defeated.

It is important you spend regular time with your cheerleaders. Cheerleaders are those people in your life who think you can do anything you set your mind to, and are excited and willing to cheer you on.

Nurturing and tending to quality relationships with loved ones helps lower our stress levels and makes us feel us more confident, optimistic and supported. When it comes to your professional goals, seek assistance and support from mentors, partners, coaches, advisors and peers. These people will help lift you to your higher potential and, if you choose carefully, will make it their mission that you succeed.

Mindful Media

Be mindful of what you are viewing, reading and listening to. When your resilience feels low, pick yourself up with a book, some music or a film about overcoming diversity.

Celebrate the Successes

As you move towards your vision, you will experience some small or large successes along the way. Acknowledge and embrace them. Consider them an indication that you are moving in the right direction and that you *can* do this!

Determination

Never give up.

ACTIVITY 1

You are filled with so many beautiful gifts and strengths. Write down everything valuable and marvellous about you. When things become stressful, bring these gifts and strengths forth. Use them to strengthen you.

_____

_____

_____

_____

_____

_____

_____

_____

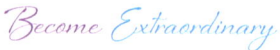

ACTIVITY 2

When things are starting to feel a little stressful in your day, grab a piece of paper. Write down all the things that are causing your anxiety or stress levels to rise. Now turn the piece of paper over and write down everything you are grateful for, everything that's going well (or even just okay), everything that makes you feel good. Now consider this. Your lists are reflective of the same life, same day, same person. Which one do you choose to focus on?

Case Study

I'd love you to meet Lily, the woman who cried for the entire two hours of our first meeting. Through her sobs, she told me she was working in a role she loved, but a recent refusal to accept the offer of a drink from her boss had transpired into her being bullied into almost submission. It was a small business and support was limited – she didn't know where to turn.

After seeking legal advice she understood her rights, but the emotional toll of her situation was proving too high and she was determined to move forward. Being stuck in a legal battle was of no interest to her. A single woman with an impending mortgage due to a recent property purchase, she was understandably afraid of losing her income. Her confidence was taking a beating. Doubt in herself and her abilities was in danger of escalating.

As she told her story, sobbing into her teacup, I could see glimpses of her strength and resilience shining through. This woman was no victim. We set to work.

Part of our plan to create her next chapter of life and career was to clarify her vision. She described a life of financial abundance, financial freedom, friendship, love, travel and independence. She no longer wanted to be at the mercy of others professionally – she wanted to start her own business and turn it into a success.

We identified her skills, strengths and gifts and brought them forth. She told me everything that was bringing her joy in her life, despite what was happening around her. We focused on cultivating her confidence and keeping the voices of doubt at bay.

Within weeks she had found the perfect part-time contract, as described in her vision, and left her current role while ensuring she received every cent she was entitled to. She had registered her business name and gathered clients without a website or any social media platforms.

Fast forward only a few years later, and she has an office, a team of people working for her, a beautiful abode and the part-time contract is a memory. Her flourishing business remains website and social media free, expanding by referral only.

Extraordinary!

Tame The Treadmill

'I respect my time more and have let go of the belief that I have to work long hours and sacrifice my personal time to prove myself.'

— Jacqui, Extraordinary Client

You get out of bed grumpy because you overslept and missed your morning workout. You wrestle with clothes that don't fit. Are they shrinking in the wash? You make a mental note to get more sleep tonight and bounce into the gym tomorrow morning.

You have a meeting with your boss who expresses yet again there is no room for movement or promotion. You are bored with this role and crave a new challenge. You know you could contribute more if only someone would give you the opportunity. If job-hunting wasn't so time consuming, you'd ditch this place for somewhere new. You wonder if you should do some further study, or find a mentor … maybe start that business you've been thinking about. But who has time?

At 2pm, you realise your healthy eating plan has flown out the window when you throw a slimy burger down your throat whilst working at your desk. You vow to yourself you will make time to pack your lunch before you leave home tomorrow.

6pm already? You race to the supermarket and throw ready-made food into a basket, silently promising yourself and your family you will leave work on time tomorrow and cook a healthy dinner from scratch.

You arrive home to a mailbox full of bills (shelve that holiday for another year, and don't even dream of those investment plans). You earn great money. Where does it go? You have no idea, and who has time to figure it out?

You welcome your partner home with a distracted peck on the cheek while pulling the kids away from the television with one hand and vacuuming with the other. You ask someone to set the table for dinner, but no one moves so you do it yourself. You do enough negotiation and conflict resolution at work and do not have the energy to do it at home, too. You wonder what's in your calendar for later this evening. Is it book club, a board meeting or a video-conference call? Or are you making cupcakes for the school fete? You're tired, irritated and fed-up. Why does it feel like you have to do *everything*?

Does this sound familiar?

When I entered my mid-forties, with fifty peeking over the horizon (eek), I began removing those things that no longer served me or my life – drama, perfectionism, excessive exercise, restrictive diets, long work hours, putting myself last, agreeing to anything that wasn't 100% Yes!

One of my favourite things to quit was using the word *busy*. I made this call when I realised that I, along with many others on the planet, was using Busy as a Badge of Honour. When did overscheduling ourselves (and often our families) become something to be proud of?

For some professionals, rushing between meetings and mock-complaining about a long task list brings forth a feeling of pride in their ability to hustle and/or their perceived importance to the organisation. We have friends who are the same, too busy for a cuppa, a walk, a catch up or a phone call.

'Hang on, Janelle!' I hear some of you protest, *'You don't know what my life/work is like. Sometimes a lot hits my plate all at once and I have to put my head down and my butt up!'* I feel you – that happens in my world as well – but there is a difference between short bursts of increased activity and long term overloading. If the rush and bustle is normal for you, your life is in danger of becoming a kaleidoscope of personal and professional commitments – a constant movement of patterns, scenes and colours you move through without really taking the time to experience or enjoy any of it. You may find yourself trapped on the treadmill.

Why do we run from one thing to another, hardly ever pausing to take a breath? Why do we feel pride in being able to 'juggle' conflicting priorities and brag about our ability to 'multitask'?

If you live solo, you may overschedule yourself due to Fear of Missing Out and/or loneliness *('is everyone else at a party right now I wasn't invited to?')* If you are a mother of an infant, it may be a desire to stay connected to life outside your familiar four walls while coping with a tiny human who is unable to engage in conversation with you. If you are career-driven, it may be the burning desire to be noticed by doing more, taking on more and never asking for assistance. If you are a parent, overscheduling your children's activities and social outings may help you feel relevant, valuable or needed.

If you are lonely or unfulfilled, no matter your situation or circumstance, remaining 'in action' distracts you from being with yourself. When you are quiet, still and reflective, the reality of your disappointing or unhappy situation – and the changes required to transform it – may feel too overwhelming and frightening to contemplate. It feels much more comfortable to stay busy and distracted, to remain in motion.

Do you have a continual need to always be surrounded by others? Do you feel the need to constantly please others? Do you dislike saying 'no' to someone?

If you answered yes to any of these questions, you may be entertaining some fear – fear of being left out of the group, fear of feeling irrelevant, fear of being left behind, fear of what others think about you, or fear of acknowledging yourself and your life in case frightening changes need to be made.

When you overcommit and find yourself feeling drained, defeated and exhausted, something has to give. Why would you stay on a treadmill that is causing damage to your physical and emotional health, your relationships and possibly your life?

Time is our only non-renewable resource. We know it's limited. We know once we use it, we never get it back. We know it's going to disappear for each and every one of us one day. So, why aren't we treating it with honour and respect? We also know time is malleable, relative to us. When we are experiencing something that brings us joy, time flies. When we are bored, it tends to pass more slowly.

Are you conscious of how you use your time? Do you allocate your time in alignment with your priorities?

If your health is your priority, do you dedicate a portion of your time to meal-plans and preparation, exercise, meditation and other modalities that support you physically, mentally and emotionally? If your family is your priority, do you allot time to family outings, school plays, junior sport, conversing and sharing meals together? If your intimate relationship is your priority, do you honour your time together by being fully present in conversations?

Or are you trapped on the treadmill of keeping your boss happy, making more and more money, proving yourself to your peers, saying yes when you want to say no, always arriving late, running from one thing to the next, snapping at your kids to hurry up, missing your yoga class, putting everyone else before yourself (and your priorities), falling into bed with exhaustion at the end of the day and pushing your partner away? Not to mention being a mediocre leader (*who has time to lead and inspire?*), the speeding fines incurred in your haste, the effect your irritability has on your relationships, your inability to sleep soundly, the unhealthy food bought and consumed on the run, the colds and flus or aches and pains that just won't seem to leave your body, and the resentment towards others that burns inside you until you explode!

Whew. Breathe! This is not what I consider *Having It All*. Living this way is a one-way ticket to *dis-ease*, in both your mind and body. And when we are in dis-ease, we are not useful to anyone, especially ourselves.

Time and energy are interlinked. Use your time wisely and you expand your energy. Use your time carelessly, you become drained and have less energy to spend doing the things in life you enjoy. No brainer, right? So why aren't you acting on it?

There's a misconception that we, as human-evolvings, are happiest lying on a beach enjoying the sunshine. Not so. As you are here, reading and working through this book, I am going to make a considered assumption you already know that to be untrue. Yes, relaxing is essential (especially if you've been disrespecting your time and energy by giving too much of it to others) and fun for a while, but you actually feel more alive when you are creatively problem solving, achieving a milestone, completing a challenge, socially and intimately connecting with others, expanding your mind, growing, creating, inspiring others and, best of all, feeling good whilst you're doing it. If this is the way *you are living your life right now, today*, take a moment to pat yourself on the back – you deserve it.

Warning: don't get too comfortable. Potential risks to your happiness are on their way, but if you're able to recognise them they won't have the power to upset your harmony.

When you are on fire in most or all areas of your life, and within yourself, two things are occurring simultaneously. Firstly, you feel fantastic – as if you can take on the world. Secondly, other people are noticing – *uh oh*. Those around you are drawn to your joyful energy and impressed by your achievements, and they want in! Your boss delegates one of her projects to you, increasing your workload. A friend inquires if you're able to collect their child from school, oh and then do you mind taking them to your place for a few hours? Your sister asks you to organise your mother's birthday party. Your partner suggests you perform more household chores because you're clearly more organised. Social and community event invitations increase as friends and associates create ways to bask in your aura.

Simultaneously, you are feeling *so energised*, empowered and motivated you say yes to every invitation and request. Before you know it you're struggling to stay afloat at work, entertaining a houseful of children, planning a party for 100, struggling through the domestic chores at home, and your calendar is booked solidly with social engagements you feel obligated to attend.

Seemingly without any conscious effort, you've found yourself back on the treadmill. All the blissful activities you were doing just for you have fallen away. You feel drained, exhausted and almost as if you are operating within a mental fog. To top things off, you've caught a damn cold that's making you feel miserable and you just can't shake it off. Insist on pushing through, and you are in danger of chronic illness, relationship breakdowns and/or burnout. *Argh!* What a rollercoaster!

Is there a way you can feel focused and motivated at work; present at home; strong and flexible in your body; calm in your mind; happy around others; at peace in yourself with enough energy to share with others purely because it brings you joy? Is it possible to create a life you don't need to take a holiday from?

Yes, there is! Let's permanently dismount from this overworked treadmill, dump it in the corner of the garage, and create a life with extraordinary energy, clear boundaries, loads of freedom and buckets of time – for yourself and whomever you choose to share it with!

ACTIVITY

Step 1

Grab a piece of paper, turn it horizontally and draw a broad arc that resembles an upside-down bell. At the far left end where the bell begins, write 'boredom/lethargy'. On the far right end where the bell ends, write 'illness/burnout'. At the very top of the upside bell (its peak), write 'energised/feeling good'.

Draw a line down the centre from the peak of the upside down bell to the bottom. This is the optimum place we, as humans being, love to be – smack bang in the middle of boredom and burnout. This is the sweet spot – when we are here we are energised, feeling good, kicking goals, creatively problem solving, feeling healthy.

Step 2

Put a mark where you feel you are sitting on that bell curve right now. Are you currently sliding down the left side of the bell, towards boredom and lethargy? Time to bring some fun and/or challenging activities into your life. Where focus goes, energy flows.

Or are you currently sliding more down the right towards illness and burnout? Time to remove things from your life, specifically things, people and places that are draining you of energy.

Are you currently rocking this life thing? Sitting at the very top? Extraordinary! List all those things, people and places you are doing or spending time with to bring you to this place. From now on, these are your non-negotiables!

_____

_____

_____

_____

_____

_____

_____

_____

Tame The Treadmill

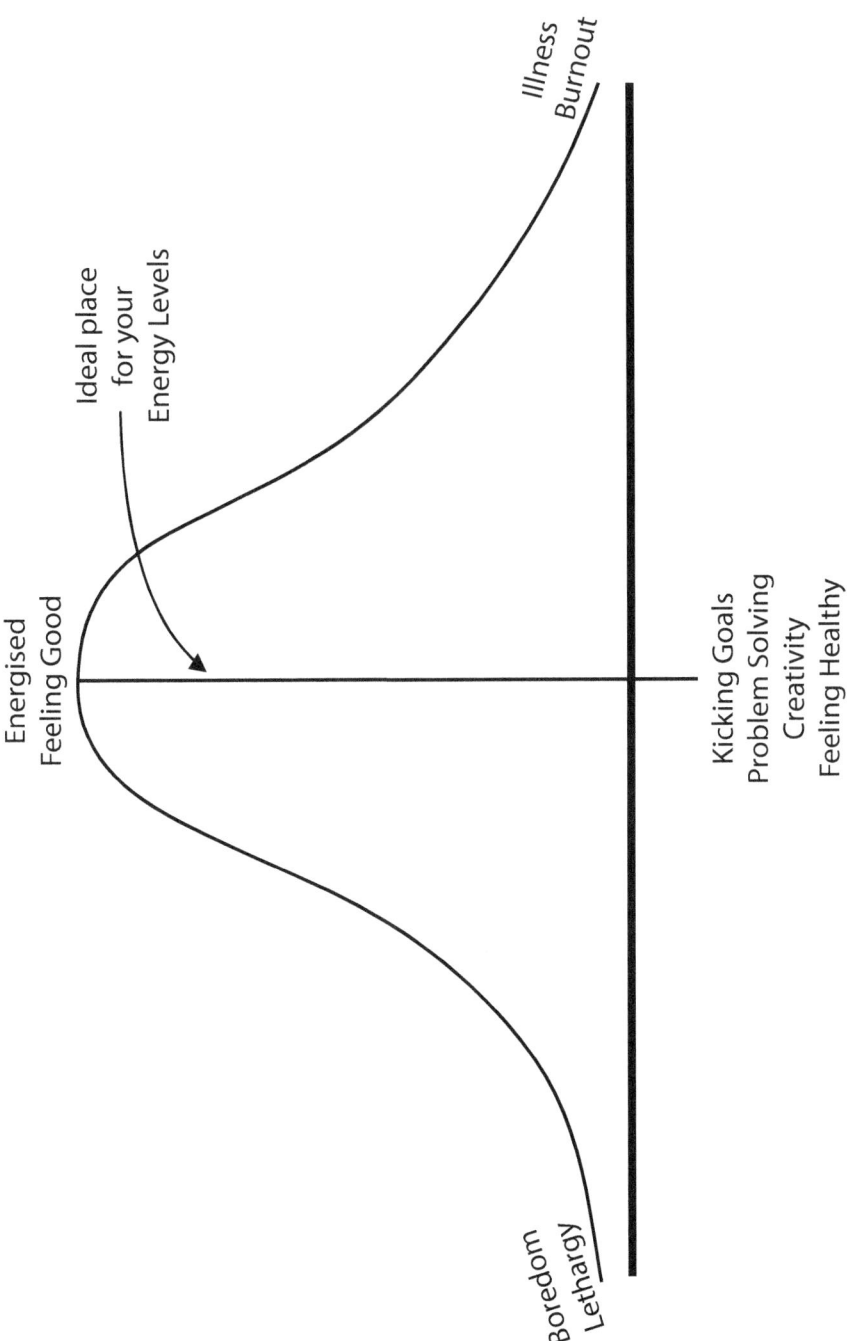

Case Study

From the outside, Dora's life looked perfect – mother of young and charismatic children, very happily married to a supportive partner, many friends, financial security, and the main breadwinner of the family via her executive role. She'd enjoyed a very happy childhood and is still close with all members of her family. To those around her, Dora Had It All. She was, they assumed, living a perfect life.

But in reality, when she came to see me, she was deeply unhappy and tumbling, at a rapid rate, down the bell curve into illness and burnout. She told me she struggled to set boundaries around her time, didn't complete things she started, felt pressured to do everything, had an inability to focus on what was important to her, felt disorganised and confused, never asked for help, tried to do too many things at once, didn't know how to enjoy life in the moment, emotionally ate, felt enslaved by perfectionism and would seek out external happiness indicators.

She admitted whilst her professional role was part-time, she often worked full-time hours. She made choices and decisions based on pleasing others, rather than herself. She took a huge breath and finished with, 'I want to let go of the 'should'. I'm so exhausted from doing things because I think I should.' She was trapped by the treadmill.

To her friends, staff, colleagues and family (the very people she was constantly needing to please) she was superwoman! But inside, she was drowning. All she wanted was to feel true, genuine and unwavering inner peace, self-love and happiness. And she was ready do the work!

Our immediate task was to identify all the people, places and activities that drained her of energy and remove them from her life, which she did courageously. Next, we uncovered which areas of her life were most important to her and deemed the top priority for her time and energy. She learned how to set boundaries around her time, say no to invitations that were not 100% Yes and communicate her needs and wants to those around her. She hit the gym, planned and prepared nutritious meals for herself and her family, began a daily meditation and gratitude practice and reintroduced long-forgotten creative pursuits that offered stillness and joy. She reduced her working hours and learned techniques to leave work in the office so she could be wholeheartedly present with her family each evening.

Recently she contacted me with the news she'd created even more time for herself and has embarked on some volunteer work for one of her favourite charities.

Dora and her life have completely transformed.

Extraordinary!

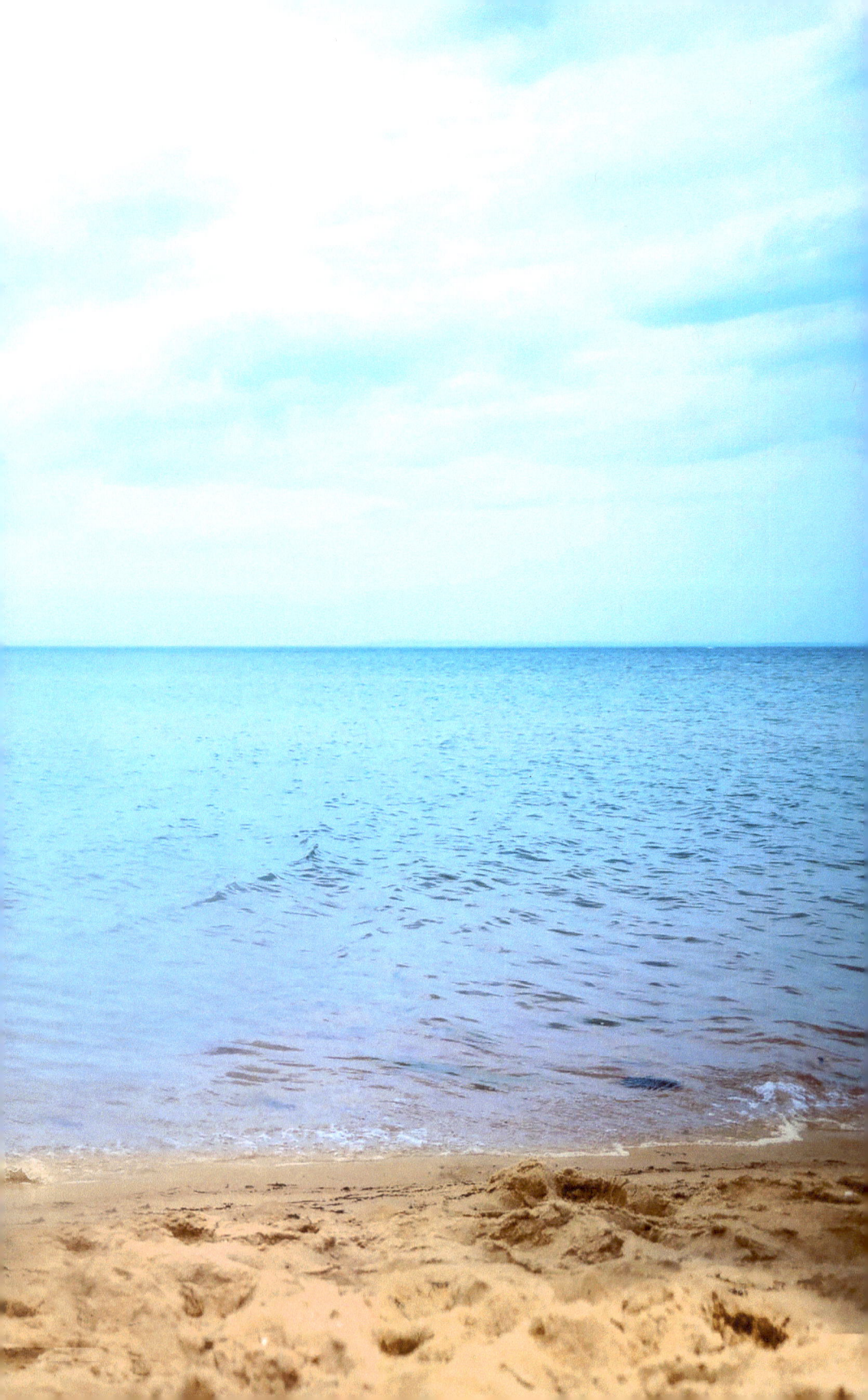

Make Friends With Fear

'I now consciously and boldly seek and step into new opportunities without fear, safe in the knowledge that I will always be okay.'

– Tamzin, Extraordinary Client

Earlier this year I was in conversation with one of my mentors and, in context with the discussion we were having, she asked me if I had a fear of success. I took my time in replying, intentionally feeling into the question. After a few moments, I told her no, I didn't believe that I had a fear of success.

Fast forward to merely weeks later (funny how life works) when I was in another conversation around fear, this time with one of my clients. To serve her in the moment, I shared a personal story of my childhood – a moment in time when I decided (due to schoolyard bullying) that to rise academically was dangerous, to excel in sport was unsafe, to raise my hand in class was perilous and to speak up was risky. In other words, I decided at a very young age that to be visible and shine my light meant losing friends and being ridiculed. It was much safer to play small, stay silent and not rock the boat. *Whoa!*

This insight inspired me to reflect over my life and pinpoint all the choices I'd made and actions I'd taken out of fear – fears I was unaware of, fears that were so discreet and so clever at hiding themselves I couldn't even recognise them when I was feeling into them!

- Resisting a professional photoshoot for, oh I don't know, years now. *Fear of spending the money, being 'too fat' for the clothes – and the potential ridicule linked to being visible.*
- Not applying for higher roles in my previous career. *Fear of not being good enough and fear of failing.*
- Resisting public speaking opportunities throughout my career. *Fear of being visible.*
- Remaining in unhealthy relationships for too long. *Fear of being single, rejected and vulnerable.*
- Dumbing myself down at secondary school. *Fear of being disliked.*
- Declining invitations to some social events. *Fear of being ignored, irrelevant or rejected.*
- Avoiding particular business networking events. *See above.*
- Use of alcohol as a crutch in certain situations. *Fear of not being good enough, rejected, ridiculed, visible.*
- Opting out of a prestigious equestrian event I'd qualified for in my teens. *Fear of not being good enough, visible.*
- Feeling anxious when sending draft chapters of this book to friends and clients for feedback. *Fear of not being good enough.*
- Staying silent when behaviour from others has been unacceptable and unaligned with my values. *Fear of rejection or upsetting others.*
- Allowing old perfectionism habits to arise so I can take 'control' of situations. *Fear of feeling vulnerable and exposed.*
- Feeling fear, in this moment, as I make this list. *Fear of being judged.*

I wanted to share these with you to remind you that no matter how you are feeling in some situations, you're not alone. I can guarantee you multiple people are feeling just as fearful, nervous and anxious as you – and they are often standing right beside you; even those you would never imagine become paralysed by fear.

I feel so sad for that *Janelle of the Past*. I feel for the little girl who stopped shining brightly, the teen who could have achieved so much more at school if she'd let herself be herself, the athlete who may have progressed further, the young woman who allowed some men to treat her so terribly (which influenced her to treat good men the same way), the professional who limited herself in her career and now the business owner who moves through the fear of being visible almost daily. But I am so happy for the Janelle who met her very first coach almost twenty years ago and has been on an adventure of self-exploration, boldness, authenticity and courage ever since.

That fact that you are reading this book, intending to expand your mind, create consciously and lead and inspire others makes me very happy, too.

What are your fears? How are they affecting your behaviours? Are you able to recognise them when they arise?

Fear is ancient. It's as old as life itself. It is an integral, profound reaction, evolved over the history of humans (and other organisms) to protect us against perceived threats to our existence. During my work and research, I've identified four types of fear:

1. Fear of Death
2. Fear of Change
3. Fear of Failure
4. Fear of Guilt

Fear of Death

Okay, so this number one fear is the Big One. This is our survival instinct coming into play, and when it does, there's no stopping it. It's powerful and primitive, and you will have no control over your mind and your body. We have this primal fear to thank for our continued existence and evolvement as a species.

Once your brain, beginning with the amygdala then backed up by the hippocampus and prefrontal cortex (the part of our brain that helps determine if the perceived threat is real), has observed a potential mortal threat, your entire system prepares to fight or flee. Copious amounts of adrenalin floods throughout your body, raising your heart rate and increasing the rate of blood flow. Your pupils dilate, your hearing becomes more enhanced. Organs not crucial to your survival slow down. This blood flows to your muscles, so they are ready to react. A current of cortisol turns fatty acids into energy (reserves so high they are usually inaccessible), for the muscles to use if required. Your muscles become tighter, causing piloerection or goose bumps. If we become trapped and unable to battle or run, we may move into a freeze response, 'playing dead' in the hope the threat will lose interest and leave.

The trigger of the perceived threat propels you into a primal, instinctive survival mode – you are on high alert to react. You are not in rational, creative or analytic thinking mode. People, post an experience of terror, have reported time slowing down, colours becoming more vivid, sounds heightened and clearer, a sense that the entire Universe is at their fingertips and a feeling of almost being superhuman. They report they did not have time (or the inclination) to 'think' about what to do next.

Many moons ago I was on a train in London on my way home from a wine-tasting event. I was with a friend, the carriage was almost empty, we were a little tipsy and looking forward to getting home. Suddenly, a man appeared in front of us. He produced a dirty linen bag and demanded we drop our money, phone, keys into the bag. In fact, that's one memory I don't think I'll ever forget – he kept chanting 'money, phone, keys, money, phone, keys'. Before I knew it, I had said *'no'* and I was laughing. It was so funny to me – I was a backpacker. I had hardly any money (and he wasn't getting what I did have), no phone (it was early 90s and, hey, backpacker), and *as if* I was going to give him my keys. I started laughing and I couldn't stop. My friend was mortified.

Our wannabe mugger, I assume utterly shocked from my response, promptly disembarked the train at the next stop and disappeared. My friend looked at me in horror, demanding to know why I'd reacted in a way that, in her mind, may have resulted in unsavoury consequences. I couldn't tell her why, because I didn't know. One theory is that I moved into *submissiveness to the object of the threat*, an aspect of the freeze response.

Fast forward to a few years later when I was robbed in Johannesburg outside the entrance of a bank. My mugger hightailed it with my credit card and the last of my cash. It happened so quickly that I cannot remember the event in detail, but unlike the situation in London I handed over my valuables – fast! My primal, instinctive fear response assessed this as a more dangerous and threatening situation and responded accordingly.

I have provided these two examples so you can clearly see how a threat perceived by the amygdala, which is then supported as real by the hippocampus and prefrontal cortex, can render us powerless over our responses. In the above situations, I was unable to think consciously, rationally, nor clearly – but I was kept alive. Definitely a fear to make friends with!

Fear of Change

Fear of change arises when we are faced with something new, different or bigger, bolder and brighter than ever before. Sometimes the change was out of our control and imposed on us, or we've decided to make a change of our own volition. Whichever path that led us to the change, we tend to feel very uncomfortable.

I think the fear of change is more aptly described as a fear of the unknown. Your mind is in charge of keeping you alive. When you're stepping into something new, different or bigger and brighter than ever before, even if you instigated the change, your mind may perceive this change as potentially dangerous.

Let's use the example of applying for a new role. Maybe you were released from your job (out of your control) or you have chosen to leave (of your own volition). As you focus on the unknown (new boss, colleagues, organisational culture and nuances of the role) your mind detects a new, unfamiliar environment on the horizon and your central nervous system prepares to step into this landscape of the unseen.

'Attention team, we have no idea what we are stepping into. Could be highly dangerous. Potentially deadly. Best brace ourselves for worst case scenario – prepare to fight, flee or freeze!'

This is why making a change, even one you've planned yourself, can be challenging. Your entire central nervous system does not support your making a change because it creates stress. It prefers your heart beating at the perfect rate, your body remaining at its optimum temperature, your blood flowing to the required organs at the necessary time, and your mind in an ideal state which is alternating between thinking, resting and engaged – whatever the situation requires at the time.

That's not to mention what has to happen to the neural pathways in your brain (the paths created by our behaviours and habits) when you make a change. When we repeatedly execute the same action, the neural pathway becomes stronger. I liken a neutral pathway to a lovely road that has been built over time in your brain, formed by the repetition of your actions. Initially it was only a track, visited once or twice. As you repeated the action, the trail became a gravel road. Over time some bitumen was laid, then some gold bricks. As it became more regularly used, lighting appeared, then maybe some pot plants along the side, followed by some trees. The more often it's used, obviously the more it's maintained.

When you decide to change the behaviour that caused the creation of this road, the 'maintenance workers' are not overly thrilled. They spent time and effort and energy on this road – they gave it all their love! And now, due to the change in your behaviour/actions/routine, it's become apparent this road is going to be left to ruin and a new one is required. More work for them to do.

Yes, conscious change is absolutely possible. People are doing it every day, but it can be a challenge when both your mind and your body are rallying against you. Don't beat yourself up if you have a slip in your resolve. Change takes time. Make friends with the fear of change. It's only trying to keep you healthy and safe when, in reality, nothing is going to mortally harm you.

Fear of Failure

You tried something and it didn't work out. That is all failure is, in a nutshell. We, as humans, have such a fear of failure because of the meaning we bequeath it. On paper, we can see how illogical, irrational and counter-productive fear of failure is, yet it can stop many of us from reaching higher, trying new things, breaking from our 'mould' and pursuing our dreams and desires – in other words, living our very best life.

We fear how others will perceive us, which originates directly from our ego. We fear what we will think about ourselves, uncertain if we will be able to process and cope with the feelings of potential disappointment, humiliation and embarrassment if we fail. We fear what will happen to us, to our dreams and even our identity if we fail. What will we do next? Who will we become?

If we were raised in a family where we were punished for failing, and we've never worked through those feelings, our fears of failure will be more significant in adulthood. If we currently work in a team or organisation that is intolerant of failure, our fear of failure may be entirely new and confined to the workplace. In its essence, fear of failure is imagining the result of a circumstance and making it negative.

What if you embraced the belief that failure is nothing more than feedback? Feedback to try again another way. Feedback that something or someone is not for you. How would it feel if you celebrated your mistakes?

I love it when I, or my clients, make a considerable balls-up, flat on our faces mistake – for two glorious, beautiful, empowering reasons:

1. That mistake was always going to happen. It was a learning experience you had to have and now it's done! It's over. It's no longer in your future, it's now in your past.

2. You learned something, and that lesson has downloaded itself into every part of your being at a cellular level. You are not the same person anymore – you have transformed. You're ready to try again or make some new choices.

Make friends with the fear of failure. It's here to serve you greatly.

Fear of Feeling Guilty

Are you someone who holds back from being, doing, having or experiencing something you desire because of perceived potential guilt?

I have some thoughts around guilt, and you can challenge me on them if you like, but I stand by them. Guilt is man-made. You were not born with guilt. It's why Toddler A can hit his playmate (Toddler B) over the head to reclaim his toy without an ounce of guilt – a toy that Toddler B stole from Toddler A in the first place, and she doesn't feel guilty either!

While it is considered an emotion, you have been taught to feel guilty. Linked to shame, we feel guilty when we think we've acted outside social norms or what is considered acceptable behaviour within the group or community we belong to. Remember that a million things had to happen, on a physical and metaphysical plane, for you to be here, and you have a divine and almighty right to be whomever you want to be and experience anything you damn well wish, no guilt necessary.

It's time to make friends with fear, because fear is such a gift! As I've shown, primitive, ancient fear will completely take over when you are threatened. This fear is automatic, instinctual, primal and uncontrollable by your conscious mind. It can save your life, which I consider to be excellent news and worth making friends with.

Our other three fears clearly tend to be limiting. What if we embraced them instead of allowing them to hold us back? What if the feeling of fear, encompassing our mind and body, is actually an indication of transformation taking place, all the way to a cellular level?

ACTIVITY

Step 1

Reflect over your life and note when you've felt absolute fear about something, but had to pop your big-person pants on and move into it. Maybe you discovered it wasn't that frightening at all.

_____

_____

_____

_____

Step 2

Reflect over your life and pinpoint those huge, mammoth mistakes, why they happened *for* you and not *to* you. What did you learn? Where was the gift?

_____

_____

_____

_____

_____

Step 3

Ask yourself some empowering questions: what would I do today if only I had a little more courage? Which fear, of the four described in the chapter, is holding me back? What is one step I can take today, to make friends with that fear so I can move forward?

_____

_____

_____

_____

Step 4

We often can't control the outcome, so consider it irrelevant. Once you've taken your step, celebrate your courage and the action you took.

_____

_____

_____

_____

Case Study

When Rachel came to work with me, she was in her mid-twenties and living her life in fear. Being the victim of quite substantial schoolyard bullying many years before had depleted her confidence in herself and her trust in anyone outside her immediate family unit. Living in her childhood home with her parents, she left the house only to fulfil her shift at a local wellness spa, then return home. Her social life was almost non-existent, as her fear of social situations rendered her powerless to interact with new acquaintances or old friends. In fact, I only met Rachel because her mother came looking for a coach and chose me.

Rachel craved friendships, a romantic relationship and a career that brought her fulfilment. With my hand on my heart, I can honestly say Rachel amazed me with her commitment to the coaching process and her courage to move from her familiar zone into the unknown. And remember the unknown was the very thing she feared the most.

Rachel and I met twice a month for six months, and the transformation within herself and her life was truly extraordinary. We worked through the process I've described above and introduced some of the tools and techniques I've outlined in other chapters of this book. Her bravery is to be applauded.

Within six months, she had reconnected with old friends and rebuilt trust; moved from her job in the wellness spa to a new more fulfilling role and started her own business.

With each small step, her fear was decreasing and her confidence flourished. I had tears in my eyes when our coaching relationship came to an end, but I knew this was just the beginning for her, and she would continue to soar.

Three years later, out of the blue, Rachel contacted me with a beautiful update on herself and her life. She had independently moved interstate for six months, without knowing anyone in the new state, which she said was the best experience of her life. Upon returning to her home town, she landed a new role she loved and had recently been promoted into a management position. She told me she'd made amazing friends; had solid supportive relationships in her life and that she was 'even putting herself out there and going on dates'.

Extraordinary!

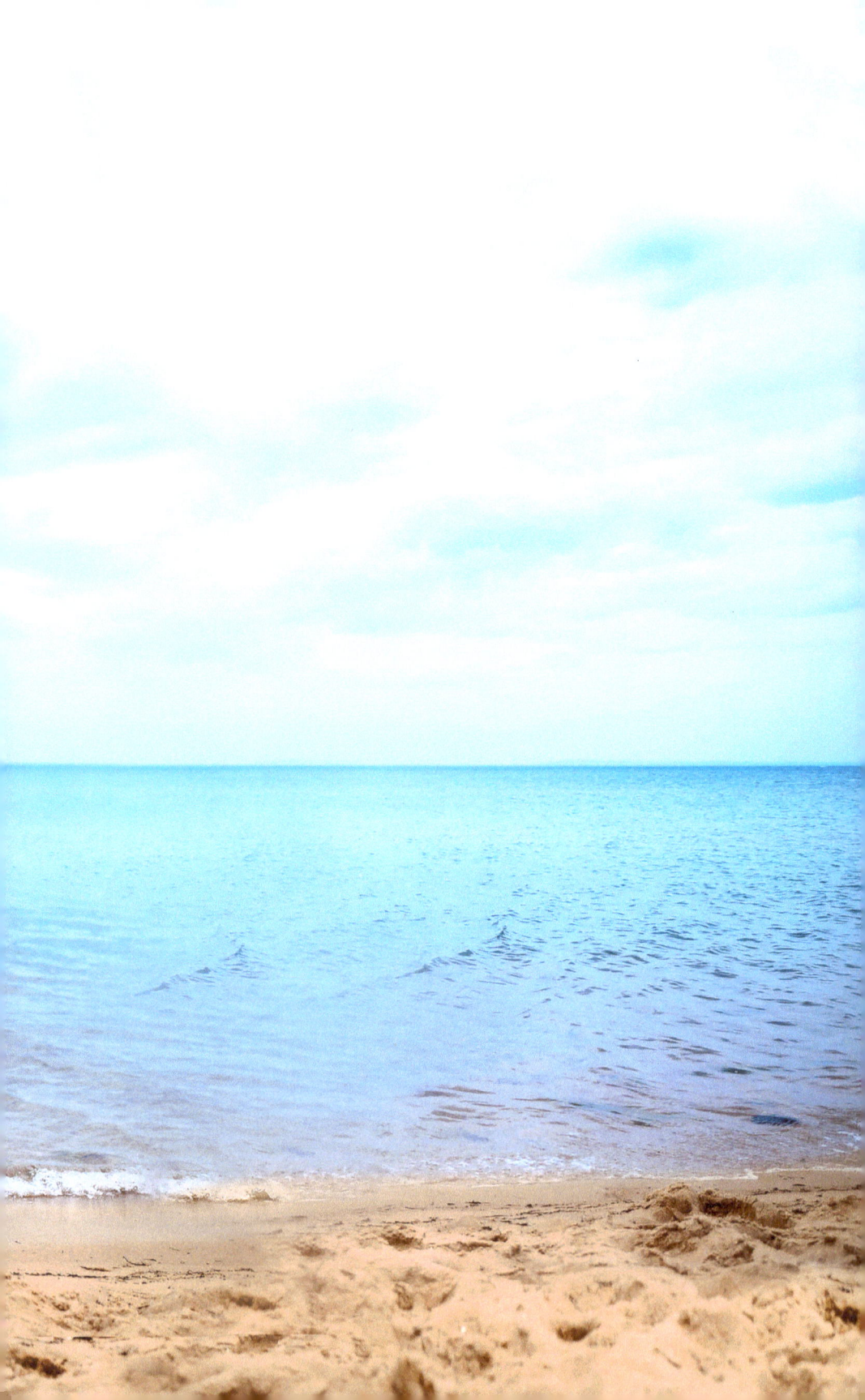

Take A Quantum Leap

'Things have happened to me that I honestly believe wouldn't have if I hadn't started on this journey. I can only imagine what else will happen as I continue to focus on quantum leaping.'

– Teena, Extraordinary Client

In an early primary school religious class, we were taught about death, heaven and hell. The teacher explained that if you were naughty or told lies, you went to hell. I told the teacher nonchalantly that hell was fine with me because all my friends would be there (not in a defiant way, just a *'logical-we-are-not-perfect'* kind of way). I went on to explain to the teacher that if I experienced death, I would unlock the secret of what happens next and could then return and share this knowledge with others. She replied that when you die, you die, and there is no coming back. I didn't believe her. *A note was sent home to my mum.*

Later in primary school, our teacher allowed us to create our very own assignment on anything we wished! As a creative and academic student, I was beyond excited and couldn't wait to get home and pull out my coloured markers and reams of paper. I wrote and illustrated a book called *The Supernatural*. Each individual page of the book introduced a supernatural or mythical being or unexplained phenomenon – from ghosts, witches and angels, to Big Foot, the Bermuda Triangle and aliens. Everyone else in my class did their assignment on their pet or family or previous holiday.

By my teenage years, I'd graduated into tarots and creating my own séances, and had developed an interest in the theory of multiple dimensions. (I have some stories that would make your hair curl!) As soon as my mother became aware of my new hobby, she put an end to it quickly! Her exact words were, *'You are messing with forces you do not understand'*. She was right.

During my years of backpacking throughout my twenties, I sought out places of wonder, curiosity and unexplained events, or historical or religious significance – areas such as Jordan, Egypt, the Dead Sea, Mount Ararat, Mount Sinai, India, Ireland, Nepal, Africa, Indonesia and Loch Ness (stared at that lake for bloody hours, willing Nessie to pop up).

From the top of the world to the bottom, I've asked people, encompassing many lands and a multitude of cultures, not only what do they *believe,* but also what do they *know*?

In my thirties I settled back in Australia and joined the corporate world. The pursuit of knowledge of the unknown dissipated, but never completely disappeared. It was reignited a few years later when I began purchasing books which introduced me to the time-space continuum and quantum physics.

Following that, when I lost my mum in 2011, I took myself off to Bali in Indonesia, one of the most significant spiritual hotspots in the world, for solitude and spiritual healing. Over one month I visited mountain temples; received blessings by shamans; experienced many profound energy healings via meditation, art therapy, chakra balancing, massage, yoga, crystal bowl healing, and a visit to one of Bali's oldest medicine men. I had some of the most incredible experiences of my life, the most enlightening being transformational breathwork.

The brochure stated this *'transformational breathwork technique directly taps you into an awareness of your essential nature and an experience of your spiritual connection'*. It was not an embellishment, and the experience did not disappoint.

Transcendental encounters are challenging to describe as they, by their very nature, remove you from the physical human existence – the realm where words exist – but I will try. I felt that my consciousness connected to, and became, 'the light' in an explosion that began by light emanating from my body – fingers and toes first, then my entire body exploding into a ball of light. I didn't have a body. I was the light – light that was endless and all-encompassing and enveloping me in pure love. I felt deeply connected to every living person and creature in the Universe, including plant life. We were all one. I felt whole. I was whisked onto this kind of cool, quick 'shoot around the Universe' ride – its purpose seemingly to prove that I was actually connected to everything.

Then I became nothing but pure consciousness and it was an incredibly blissful experience. While I stayed locked in this moment, unencumbered by a physical body or any time construct, I received messages about myself, my life, the man I'd just met (now Handsome Hubby) and members of my family. I was told I was full of light and love and to stop being afraid; to stop being so fearful of what other people thought of me; that my life is how it's supposed to be; to never worry about money as I will always have as much as I need; I will always be taken care of; to not worry about the type of work I do as long as I do it out of love and passion, not money to appease my ego. Then white light swirled around my hip and knee, where I was carrying small injuries at the time, and it was over.

Although I was physically depleted and highly emotional for hours afterwards, it was such an extraordinarily joyful experience that I wanted to do it all again the next day! I truly believe I was given a glimpse of what's on the 'other side', as per my childhood request. I now feel it's up to me to honour my side of the agreement – that I would return and share what I know.

Upon my return home from Bali, my desire to learn more about the magical grew from an ember back into a flame, and I immersed myself in learning more about who we are, why we are here, and how the Universe works on both a spiritual and scientific level.

Everything is made of energy, including us. I don't need science to tell me that – I have personally experienced it. What if we were always in flow, never out of flow? What if we could use the basic principles of quantum physics to step into a new dimension of our life? How would that be possible? Is pushing and striving until we burn out the only road to 'success'? Or is there another way that feels more elegant and graceful and joyful? If so, how do we tap into that? And what is 'success' anyway?

It is scientifically proven that humans emit energy. What if we used that energy more efficiently? And how do our thoughts affect our energy? What happens to the energy we emit into the world? How does it affect our families and colleagues and community, if at all?

What is time? Can we create more of it for ourselves? What if we teamed this with mastery of our minds, conscious and subconscious? How can we use this knowledge to create whatever it is we desire? If we are energetic entities having a physical experience, how do we bridge the spiritual and the material?

So many questions and so much to learn. I have to tell you, I've had so much fun reading, asking, conversing, experimenting, listening, analysing and diving into natural laws, spiritual laws, physics and universal energy! I have reams of paper with handwritten notes, multiple journals which helped me make sense of the musings in my mind and hundreds of Word documents I used to bring it all together. There is so much information that, honestly, it would take another book to share it all with you.

But I'm not going to leave you hanging – I wouldn't do that. I am going to share with you a simple concept which has the power to change your life in ways you've never imagined.

The concept is *increasing your energetic vibration to a level that corresponds with the energetic vibration of whatever you wish to do, be, have or experience in your life.* What is the simplest, easiest and fastest way to raise your vibration? Here are two ways that I've found highly successful, as have my clients – Gratitude and Visual Mental Rehearsal.

Gratitude

Let's leap into the power of appreciation – gratitude. Part of my research over the past decade involved speaking with women of the world who were successfully living their passion and purpose. I wanted to know exactly how they moved from struggle or self-doubt into success. For approximately two years, I connected with hundreds of women and asked them the same five questions. The participants included women I already knew, and women referred to me by other women. (Women shining the light on other women made my heart sing).

The pool of participants was extremely diverse and included various nationalities, religions, ages and occupations. I spoke with social warriors, professionals, creatives, entrepreneurs, solopreneurs, elite athletes, artists, award winners and quiet achievers. We connected in-person, via phone or video-conferencing. I recall one conversation with a woman in Hong Kong spanning three hours, and another that took ten minutes. As I recall how generous they were with their time, knowledge, insights and secrets, I can feel my gratitude and appreciation vibrating in this very moment.

As mentioned earlier, I was very interested in any setbacks or obstacles they had incurred during their adventure, how they had overcome them and the main factors that had contributed to their success. What was at the crux of their turning point? Was it one thing, or multiple? Did they just get lucky?

The most common reply was *'gratitude'*. These extraordinary women explained that as soon as they started to practise gratitude for opportunities, soulmate clients, grants received, super-star employees and other good fortune – no matter how small or seemingly irrelevant – everything came together for them in beautiful and graceful ways they could not have imagined. It appeared as though the moment they felt grateful for something, it generated a roll-on affect and they received more to be thankful for!

Great. Now we know how to receive anything and everything we've ever desired. Send out a bucket of gratitude. Easily done!

For some, however, this is not so easy at all – especially if everything in your creative pursuit, business, career, health, passion project or, hey, maybe your entire life appears to have gone down the toilet. But this one little practice does have the power to turn everything around.

I invite you to bring to mind a moment you did something thoughtful for someone else and they did not say thank you, they were not grateful. How inspired were to you to repeat the action?

Now bring to mind a moment you did something thoughtful for someone else and they were very appreciative. How inspired were you to repeat the action?

If you can close your eyes and imagine something (anything!) that you love in your life, you have the ability to practise gratitude. When you are in a state of gratitude that encompasses thought, feeling and emotion, you are sending out a signal to the Universe that says *'Thank you so much, I'd love some more to be grateful for, please'*.

Visual Mental Rehearsal (VMR)

The second most accessible and effective way I've found to raise my energetic vibration to a level that connects me to new experiences I desire is by practising Visual Mental Rehearsal (VMR). If you've been playing along with me since the beginning of this book, you've not only tried this, you are practising it every day through *conscious creation*. I wonder, what have you manifested into your life already?

Let's leap into how VMR works. Your mind does not know the difference between imagining something and experiencing something. This is why a memory, sad or joyful, creates a strong emotional response in your body. When you bring a memory forward, your mind assumes it is experiencing the event *in real time* and your body responds by creating the feeling or emotion that aligns with the event.

The feeling or emotion then drives your actions – the choices and decisions you make in that moment. If you are waking up every day with the same thoughts, and thus emotions, as yesterday, then it makes sense that you are repeating the same choices and taking the same actions. If the thinking that got you *here* is not the thinking that will get you *there*, then it's time to change your thinking.

What if, upon waking each day, you practised VMR by focusing on what it is you wish to create in your life? If you can bring that vision to life, using all your senses, if you can see, smell, hear, taste and touch it, your mind thinks that event is happening and sends the signals to your body to produce the corresponding emotions.

And if your emotions drive your actions, doesn't it make sense that you are more likely to make new and different choices and take new actions? Actions that are more aligned, and more likely to lead you towards and into your vision?

Set an intention to practise Visual Mental Rehearsal daily and you will feel more excited about your day and your future. You will be more inspired to move into your vision *that very same day,* as if there is no passage of time required. And if you are feeling more inspired and confident that you are consciously creating your vision, here and now today, you will move through your day feeling *oh-so-grateful* for a vision that is under creation with the same vibrational frequency as if it was already here – for the life of freedom and abundance (health, wealth and happiness) that you desire and deserve unfolding before you. We've just learned that practising *gratitude* is the greatest factor to opportunities presenting themselves as if by magic.

My challenge to you is, once you've entered this highly vibrational state, the state you've risen to from practising gratitude and imagining that your vision is already your reality, is to keep it at that level throughout the day, every day. *This is the key.*

If you reflect over your life you may see that everything you've created of value has been created from this state of being – a state of joyfulness, happiness, gratitude, clarity, excitement, optimism, energy, confidence, love and often a deep inner knowing. This is a very empowering state to live in and create from.

Alternatively, when we allow something or someone external to us bring us down we fall into a state of discomfort or suffering. When in this state, we feel fearful, doubtful, confused, irritated, annoyed, frustrated, defeated, angry, sad and drained of energy. This is a very disempowering state to live in and attempt to create from.

Take a moment to consider this – you are always operating from one state or the other. In every moment of every day, you are either in joy or in suffering. You can't simultaneously have one foot in one and one in the other.

If we create things of value in our lives from a place of gratitude, joyfulness, happiness and optimism, doesn't it make sense to generate that feeling and remain there for as long as we can? Of course! But remember we are human-evolvings, not machines, designed to feel a range of emotions. We are built to feel sadness and disappointment at times. The trick is being able to move from a state of suffering back to a state of joy anytime you choose. How? By recognising and understanding your emotions, naming them, working through them and harnessing them or releasing them.

Once you've mastered the concept of *increasing your energetic vibration to a level that corresponds with the energetic vibration of whatever you wish to do, be, have or experience in your life,* you unlock unseen forces around you that are waiting to serve you.

These forces are larger than any macro or micro obstacle you can imagine and they are always in play. You have the ability and opportunity to move from your three-dimensional reality into the quantum, the realm of never-ending possibility. You are ready, and poised, to take a quantum leap.

Quantum Theory

Quantum theory is the study of how the world works at a subatomic level and has been referred to as the *physics of possibility*. It's whacky, fun and mind boggling and takes a little to wrap your head around, but it's also very exciting.

Quantum experiments discovered that everything in the Universe, including us, is made up of energy and matter; the ratio being 99.99% energy and, the rest, matter. Energy is frequency and all frequency emits and receives information. Quantum theory also tells us this energy or frequency has consciousness, so everything in the Universe, including us, is 99.99% energy and consciousness and that a very small part is matter.

This field of consciousness is referred to as the quantum field or realm, and we, as vibrational beings, vibrate in and out of this field multiple times per second. This field of consciousness is filled with information or, if you prefer, *all possibility and potentiality*. Quantum theory proves nothing is separate to us – everyone and everything is connected via a field of consciousness. The quantum pioneers thought this was very cool – they wondered then, if we are almost pure consciousness, if we enter and exit this field of all possibility and potentially multiple times throughout our day, are we able to return from the field with a new experience? And can we bring that experience into our lives immediately? Instantly?

This brings us to another weird and wonderful finding of quantum physics – that you cannot undertake a quantum experiment without an observer. Quantum scientists discovered that particles can also act like waves (of energy) and when observed they are almost forced to behave like particles. When unobserved they collapse back into waves. Whilst they found the behaviour of the particles to be unpredictable, the probable outcome was the one they were looking for.

By now, you are most likely starting to wonder what this all has to do with you and your life. The physics lesson is over. Let's not talk about quantum leaping anymore, I prefer to put it into practise. Allow me to show you how it works.

You are now aware you are a vibrational being (your body is made up of approximately 50 million cells and each cell generates around 1.4 volts of electricity, which means there's about 700 trillion volts of electricity in your body right now), and that your being vibrates out of a field of consciousness where all possibilities and potentialities await you.

You are now aware that you create things of value (bring them back with you from the field) when you are crystal clear on what you wish to experience – your vision – then *feel deep, overwhelming and heartfelt gratitude* for it. Those emotions drive us to make new choices and take aligned action. Quantum physics tells us that particles collapse into waves until they are observed. When they are observed they become matter – in other words, they appear in your reality.

So my questions to you are: what are you observing? What are you focused on? Are you focused on heartbreak, bad 'luck', illness, an empty bank account, a lacklustre career, a failing business? Are you focused on past events and circumstances that caused you suffering, and allowing those memories to hold you back in the present and hinder your future?

Let's revisit what I experienced that first time in my pure state of consciousness in Bali:

- No time
- No body
- No thing
- Pure love
- Pure energy
- Ray of light
- Expansion
- Limitlessness
- Connectedness to everyone and everything
- Message to release fear
- Message to release worry
- Message to live for joy and passion (not money or ego)

Making your Quantum Leap

What if we could enter the quantum realm and pick out the very things we wish to be, do have and experience, then watch them manifest (appear) in our lives, as if by magic? We can, and plenty of people already do.

You may hear it referred to as taking a Quantum Leap – a leap that is easy, effortless, graceful and time-saving; one of exponential rather than incremental progress; and is often a move that makes zero sense until after the fact.

To gain a sense of what this means, here is something I was once shown by a mentor. Stand up and focus on a place on the floor about an arm's length in front of you. While focusing on that exact spot, jump and land directly on it. Excellent, good leaping!

What were you focused on when planning to jump? The spot on the floor, right? What were you focused on as you jumped? Most likely, you were still focused on the spot on the floor, as you simultaneously sent an instructional signal to your legs (to take action, to move).

What were you focused on while you were in the air? I'm going to guess, still the spot on the floor – or, in other words, the place you wanted to land! You chose your destination (the spot on the floor), took action (emitted energy to jump) and landed precisely where you put your focus.

There was no energy wasted on worrying about being in the air, what could go wrong in the air, if you were worthy enough to be in the air, what others would think about you being in the air, if you were actually qualified or if you were good enough to be in the air. You leapt with absolute faith that you would land safely at your pre-determined destination.

Quantum leaping is the act of transitioning from one place to another, without the step-by-step process to do so. And this is so freaking exciting to me, I can feel my heart rate increasing and my vibration rising just as I write this sentence. All the cells in my body are tingling in an excellent way. Can you feel the freedom this brings? The empowerment this brings?

You are not your past.
You are not your memories.
You are not your parents.
You are not your current status-quo.
You can make a quantum leap at any time.

But you have to be willing to take the risk. You have to be willing to step away from conventional thinking. You have to be willing to take the ride, go on the adventure and be ready to do things in possibly the opposite way you've done them before. I am going to leave you here, with some of the principles of quantum leaping.

As you move through this activity you may notice we are bringing everything together, everything you've learned, from the moment you picked up this book. Thank you for being here, for choosing me to be by your side as you expanded you mind. I've had so much fun with you, and hope you have already begun to see how extraordinary you are.

Are you ready to take your next leap? You've got this!

Principle 1
Expand Your Mind To New Ways To Succeed

When we achieve success, as a direct result of specific behaviours, we tend to repeat those behaviours to obtain even more success. Those behaviours become familiar and we will keep repeating them, even when we do not see desired results.

A quantum leap requires taking a new risk – trying something different, and exploring the unconventional.

Action: *What new, seemingly risky or unconventional behaviours could you implement today?*

PRINCIPLE 2
Remove Your Blinkers

Release the conventional 10-step plan. A quantum leap requires taking one step, then opening your eyes to the new opportunities and possibilities in front of you. It's from here, this place, you decide on your next step.

Action: *What is your very next step towards your vision? What ideas do you have that you have yet to try?*

Principle 3
Create Some Space

If what you are doing isn't working, stop doing it. Even if you are unsure what do to instead, giving yourself some mental space and physical time will allow new inspiration and ideas to fly in. Quantum leaps require doing something new, something that is elegant, graceful and simple.

Action: *What habits and routines are preventing you from stepping into your vision? What can you stop doing today?*

Principle 4
Become Limitless

Switch your focus from blocks, obstacles and restraints and turn it to your desired creation – the destination! You were born with limitless power, energy and potential. Decide what you want, then times it by ten or one hundred or one thousand! Achieving this will require an expansion of your mind – breaking free from old conditioning, self-limiting beliefs and constraints. Give your soul permission to soar! A quantum leap requires uncommon sense.

Action: *Revisit your vision. Does it require updating? Expansion?*

_____

_____

_____

_____

_____

_____

_____

_____

Principle 5
Act with Certainty

Release any fear and doubt and act as though your success is guaranteed. Practise unwavering faith and trust in yourself and the process. Do what you would do, act how you would act, behave how you would behave if success was certain. A quantum leap requires being bold.

Action: *After focusing on your vision each day, set an intention for yourself. What actions would you take today if your success was certain?*

PRINCIPLE 6
Focus on Your Destination

If you ever worked with me, this line will be very familiar to you: you don't need to know how you're going to get there, but you need know where 'there' is.

A quantum leap requires Visual Mental Rehearsal. Decide where you want to land and focus on your arrival. It's not your job to worry about how. Stay open, present and listen – the answers will come to you. All the resources you require are already here. A quantum leap is not something you design and orchestrate – you just allow it to happen. A quantum leap requires accepting some disorder and confusion without a plan – the plan will unfold as you go.

Action: *How will you ensure you focus on your Vision at least once per day, in a way that raises your vibration to an optimum level?*

PRINCIPLE 7
Embrace the Mystical

We didn't invent electricity, we discovered it. Do you know how it works? I don't. Do you use it to your benefit? Me too! Forces are working all around us that we cannot see. Quantum leaps require a mixture of Visual Mental Rehearsal, raised vibration, guidance from your intuition and, well, magic. Remain focused on your destination, move towards it with confidence and watch the forces align and work for you.

Action: *Become more aware of synchronicities and coincidences, by creating a 'The Magic I Saw Today' evening practice. Before you retire to bed in the evening, make a list of all the synchronicities, coincidences or 'lucky breaks' you experienced that day. This activity will awaken you to the magic that's unfolding every day.*

Principle 8
Give Yourself a Chance

Right now, taking a quantum leap may feel like an enormous risk. But what is the risk of remaining in the status quo? The risk of not reaching your potential? Not fulfilling your dreams?

A quantum leap requires challenging your limits, challenging the odds and moving out of your familiar zone. Expand your mindset. Challenge your unhelpful thoughts. Embrace the opportunity you've been avoiding.

Action: *Complete this sentence: 'This is the risk of NOT moving into what I want...'*

PRINCIPLE 9
Take Action

I've never believed we can stare at a pretty picture of an object we desire and have it appear in front of us. I do believe the Universe will assist us, but meets us halfway. We need to make the first move. Wishing and hoping is not creating. A quantum leap requires pursuit.

Action: *What would I do today if I called on a little more of my courage?*

PRINCIPLE 10
Prepare to Fail

If a quantum leap requires a new way of thinking and the implementation of new behaviours, you are most likely going to experience some trial and error. Mistakes and setbacks are part of trying something different. They are not a signal to quit – they are stretching your capabilities.

Action: What will I think, say and do when I experience a setback?

Principle 11
Get Comfortable Feeling Uncomfortable

Taking a quantum leap will render you feeling freaked out, nervous, fearful, uncomfortable or all of the above. As I've clearly outlined throughout this book, transformation is impossible without moving out of your familiar zone. If you are levelling-up your thoughts, changing your behaviours, calling on courage and moving into the unknown, you are going to be challenged by your old beliefs and limitations. A quantum leap requires continuing towards your vision, despite these feelings.

Action: When was the last time I felt truly uncomfortable about an action I took and what was the result? What did I learn from this experience?

PRINCIPLE 12
Don't Delay

A quantum leap is not about waiting until your proverbial ducks are all in a row or you feel ready. Remember, a quantum leap requires you to move before you feel ready, as if your success is already absolute. It is already a step you're prepared to make – you just haven't made it yet.

Action: What action have I been procrastinating on? What is the benefit of taking that action today?

Principle 13
Trust Yourself

Every resource you'll ever need is already here, within you and around you. By now, I hope you absolutely understand how we create our world from the *inside out*.

Action: Reflect over your life and pinpoint those times you wholeheartedly backed yourself. What was the result? What did you learn about yourself?

Acknowledgements

Writing a book is a lot more challenging that I thought it would be. I take my hat off to anyone and everyone who has ever put pen to paper with no other agenda than to serve others. The world is a better place because of your commitment and dedication.

To Kate James; thank you for being the very first coach who saw something within me that I could not, and for spending the time to bring it forth. Every moment spent with you is of value, and those snippets of time, in your home nursing cups of herbal tea, transformed me and my life. Thank you for writing the foreword for this book. I am forever grateful to you. I wonder if Sky High Coaching, or this book, would exist if I had not met you.

I thank all the teachers, mentors and coaches who came afterward. In particular, the following: Rich Litvin; you accepted a new coach from Australia into your world-renowned program and showed me my power – thank you for seeing me. Giovanna Capozza; you invited me to co-create an international retreat with you, which turned out to be an incredibly life-changing experience. Your coaching abilities are first class and I learned so much from you. Thank you for still today being one of my greatest teachers and cheerleaders. Hayley Carr; we bonded over sport, travel, business, cups of tea and a desire for deep conversation – thank you for asking me the tough questions, lifting the veils I hid behind and always loving me fiercely.

Thank you Lisa Cavill, Wendy Barron, Stephanie Abouatallah, Giovanna Capozza, Sidonie Berke, Nikki Karpeles, Jacqui Lang, Madeline Knight, Melissa Delaney, Alicia Dumais Temmerman, Hayley Carr, Christine Warren, Stella Seed, Sarah Antwerpes and Meagan Solomon for reading draft pages and providing your thoughts.

Thank you Madeline Knight, Peter Dawidowski, Gabrielle Costin, Jacqui Lang, Tamzin McLennan, Teena Finch, Katie Beattie, Stephanie Abouatallah and Sidonie Berke for gifting me your inspirational quotes.

Thank you Lisbeth Mudge, Alison Wood and Eva Brookes for editing my initial musings all those years ago. Without those baby steps, and your support during the process, I may not have found the courage to write an entire book.

Thank you to everyone at Busybird Publishing for bringing this book to life in all its colour and beauty. Blaise van Hecke, this book would not have seen the light of day without your gentle encouragement and expert advice, thank you. Meg Hellyer, the super editor. Thank you for truly taking the time to get to know me and my book. Thank you for your insightful suggestions, extraordinary proofreading skills and your patience. Kev Howlett, thank you for the images and creating such a beautiful cover. Thank you Natalie Rowe for capturing the essence of me through your camera lens – you are a gorgeous soul who left us too soon – rest in peace.

Huge thanks to my family: Brian Farley, Kelvin Farley, Allison Farley, Liam Farley, Emma Farley, Jocelyn Ryan, Joy Mills, Alan Mills, Aidan Mills, Connor Mills and Alanna Mills for never-ending words of encouragement, support and glasses of wine.

Acknowledgements

To the big, colourful, vibrant, loud, elegant assortment of fabulous people in my life – my clients – my gratitude for you is all-encompassing. You are all inspiring, courageous and extraordinary. Thank you for choosing me to share your dreams, fears and secrets with. I am truly honoured.

To all my friends, from far and wide, who have supported me throughout the writing and publishing process: my deepest thanks. In particular, Sue Wilkinson, your steadfast belief in me has been pivotal in the creation of this book; Karen Pattullo for constant encouragement via email and Zoom; Melissa Delaney for brainstorming and sharing of ideas; Natalie Fisher for walks, wine, facemasks and putting my stories before her own; Alison Wood for being my sounding board during endless laps of Balwyn; Eugenie Douglas, who requested weekly updates during bootcamp, and Lisa Cavill, purely for her excitement and enthusiasm; *'is it ready yet?'*

Ziggy, you were easily my best stress release and cure for writer's block. Thank you for the cuddles and play!

To Brianna and Jon Ryan, thank you for your continual support – closed doors, muted TV, cooked dinners and a packed dishwasher. You two are the best and I love you both.

To the love of my life, Marty Ryan. Marty, for almost ten years you've sacrificed so I can achieve my dreams. I am so proud to call you my husband. Thank you for your unwavering belief in me and for your love and support, especially when I'm feeling stressed and it emerges as grumpiness. That must be why you've spent so much time lately in the brewery. Your beer certainly tastes good! Love you HH.

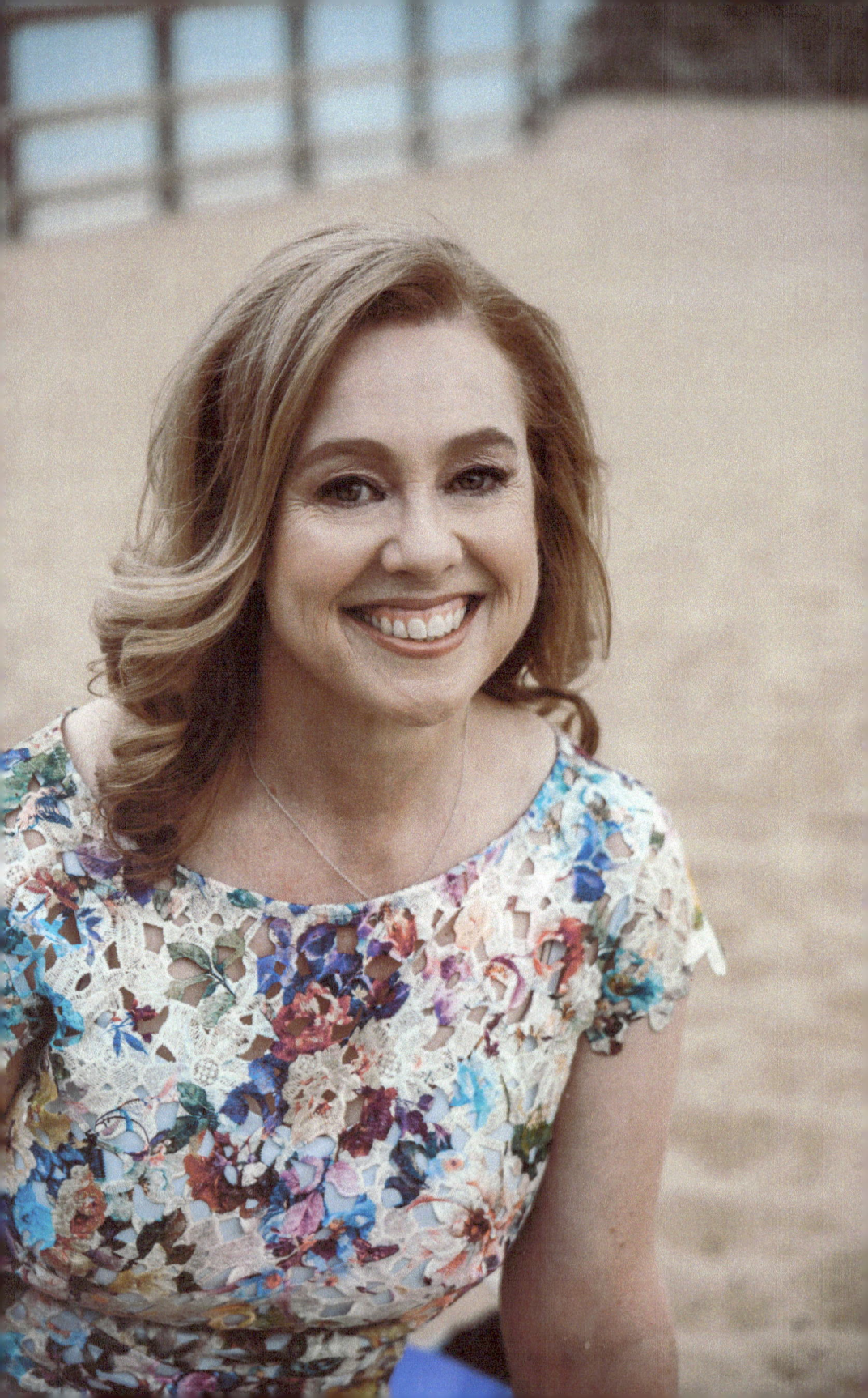

About The Author

Janelle Ryan is an award-winning global personal coach and founder of Sky High Coaching. She is also a published author, international retreat leader, workshop facilitator and inspirational speaker.

She was named one of Australia's Top 10 Female Entrepreneurs by *My Entrepreneur Magazine* in 2017.

Janelle helps high performers create extraordinary lives. Her clients include professionals, executive and emerging leaders, entrepreneurs, business owners, elite athletes and creatives! Janelle's passionate and enthusiastic nature, along with her unwavering belief in her clients, makes her a natural in helping people who are ready to take their careers, businesses or lives to the next level.

Since founding Sky High Coaching, Janelle has delivered programs and individual coaching to organisations across the finance, recruitment, tourism, sport (management and coaching), energy, legal, technology, real estate, event, government and education industries. Companies such as Google and Pullman Hotels Worldwide have entrusted her to coach their teams and individual employees to success.

She has a gift of seeing behind the facade and bringing forth her clients' true innermost skills, strengths, and desires – even those they are not necessarily aware of themselves.

Janelle believes the path to a fulfilling and blissful life and career is not merely about goal setting and achievement. Nor does it require pushing harder, working longer, or piling more onto our plate. She believes underlying the pursuit of every goal is the need to make the change required – this change could be physical, mental, emotional, or relational and can often be made with elegance and ease.

Janelle works with her clients on clarifying their vision, creating a strategy to achieve it, sharpening their emotional intelligence, busting through their self-doubt and creating the confidence required to step into a life of joy, energy and fulfilment.

A natural at working with others, Janelle finds that personal, private one-on-one coaching feeds her soul, and she loves nothing more than the time she spends with clients from 6 to 12 months.

Her second great love is her group coaching salon, which brings together a group of extraordinary like-minded souls who nurture and support each other as they work towards the creation of their personal vision.

For clients who prefer self-paced, online coaching, she offers two online programs, 'Taking The Leap' and 'Becoming Extraordinary', where she has the joy of seeing her gorgeous online community group consciously create truly Extraordinary lives!

To learn more about Janelle and her current programs, visit her website at **www.skyhighcoaching.com.au**.

To receive your thank you gift for purchasing this book, email **janelle@skyhighcoaching.com.au** and mention this offer.